Take My Hand

Take My Hand

THE CAREGIVER'S JOURNEY

TAKE MY HAND

THE CAREGIVER'S JOURNEY

Tia Amdurer, LPC
Reflections by Chris Renaud-Cogswell

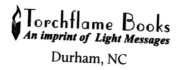

Torchflame Books
An imprint of Light Messages
Durham, NC

Take My Hand: The Caregiver's Journey
Tia Amdurer, LPC
www.takemyhandjourney.com
TakeMyHandJourney@gmail.com

Published 2018, by Torchflame Books
an Imprint of Light Messages
www.lightmessages.com
Durham, NC 27713 USA
SAN: 920-9298

Paperback ISBN: 978-1-61153-272-2
E-book ISBN: 978-1-61153-271-5
Library of Congress Control Number: 2017963114

The reflections and journal anecdotes are written by and used by permission of Chris Renaud-Cogswell.

CONTENTS

PREFACE

If you have picked up this book you probably are caring for a loved one or know someone who is. As the baby boomer generation moves into the twilight years and as life expectancy increases, more and more Americans will be caring for their elders. While homecare had been the stated choice for previous generations ("You must promise never to put me in a nursing home!"), the proliferation of retirement communities, senior care centers and memory care facilities, tells us that while there may be more choices for living options, chances are at least one sibling or relative will be caregiving in some capacity.

Giving care and being the responsible party for a parent or parents can be one of the most stressful times in an adult's life. For many in the "sandwich generation," this means juggling a career, children, perhaps grandchildren, and elders who rely on you. Often lost in this turmoil is the emotional health of the caregiver. This book is designed to help transform the caregiver's pain and powerlessness into healing, hope, and growth.

The journey every person walks is totally unique, but there is collective wisdom to help you navigate your path.

A phrase I often use as a grief counselor and bereavement specialist: this is a bittersweet time. I have learned that in spite of the sorrow, there is great tenderness and remarkable honor in hearing the stories of the journey. In the same vein, the trials and tribulations of a caregiver can be incredibly rewarding. We each get back so much more than we give—the stories of a lifetime, being present to heartbreak and healing, laughing through the tears. Laughter is a necessary component of healthy healing, so this book approaches the end of life care with humor.

When my friend Chris began sharing through social media her personal story of her aging parents and then specifically her journey with her mom, I saw her authentically exposing her raw emotion. There was such honesty and wit in her writing that I wanted to bring her experience to a wider audience. I laughed and I cried reading her posts. I hope you will too.

Contributor Chris Renaud-Cogswell is a creative, enthusiastic piano teacher with a passion for working with students with special needs. It was Chris's writing that sparked the development of this book. As a loyal daughter, Chris took on the caregiving role for her ailing parents, Esther and Bill in their late 80s. She and her devoted husband Kevin shared with her parents the transitions from parental home to assisted living community, rehab facility, and finally home and hospice care. She shared her honest and eclectic view on life with her friends and family on social media. Chris states her greatest joys include "playing with her grandchildren, cooking way too much food for family gatherings, taking an excessive amount of photos of her cat, and playing Candy Crush."

As a Licensed Professional Counselor, I find great comfort and fulfillment working in the bereavement field and holding sacred space for those who are grieving. I have years of therapeutic work in hospice and private practice, specializing in healing from loss as well as working with those suffering the scars of abuse and neglect. I enjoy doing play therapy with kids and "therapizing" with teens and adults. Creating healing rituals is a favorite technique of mine.

Many personal experiences have gone into my own understanding of end-of-life journeys—the hospice death of my dear cousin, and traumatic deaths of my nephew, uncle, and brother-in-law. I was a caregiver for my father-in-law and a long-distance support for my sister as she cared for my parents.

How to Use This Book ...

Know that we use the term "parent" throughout the book, but we are approaching caregiving as a specific experience whether for a parent, relative, spouse, friend or sibling. Of course, the losses are different. But individuals each grieve differently and each bereavement is unique, so we hope you will relate to the issues and fill in your own blanks.

Since every end-of-life is special, you may find yourself drawn to certain chapters at different times; there is no wrong way to read this book. We have ordered this book by topics rather than chronologically. Chris's writing is in a distinct font showing her vulnerability, frustration, love, and humor as she cared for her mom and dad. My narratives include ways you might experience your own situation and suggest some therapeutic alternatives. Finally, at the end of each chapter, is a page for you to reflect on your journey. The relationship you and your loved one have is likely complicated. As you journey together down this uneven path, take time now and then to find some stillness and recognize your own worth.

One of the most comforting yet painful moments in my life will forever be the time I heard my mother call out, "Mom? ... " when she needed to use the bathroom ... We call out, "Mom?" and we know everything will be okay. We say, "Mom?" and our shoes will be tied, our boo-boos will be kissed, our tummies will be filled ... We call out, "Mom?" and we know we will soon be warm, we will be caressed, we will be loved. Mom?

ACKNOWLEDGMENTS

From Tia ...

There are always those who support and encourage you as you take on important projects—some make constructive criticism, others provide cheerleading from the side. Still others in this virtual village send loving thoughts from beyond.

In the here-and-now, I want to express my gratitude to my husband Michael Amdurer for his patience and support; my son Zach Amdurer, PA-C, for his medical stamp of approval, his jazz, and his delight in learning something new; my daughter, Francesca Kühlers, for the eagle eyes of a copy-editor; and sisters Laura Minor and Jeanne Buesser for their encouragement and our forever-bond. On the editing side, Wally Turnbull from Light Messages believed in the worth of this book and provided guidance, Kevin Cogswell offered careful review, Lois Feinstein provided talented oversight, and editor Milton Brasher-Cunningham just rocks.

To expand my knowledge, I relied on the expertise provided by Robin Jamison, LCSW, a professional artist and End-of-Life doula. Her journey with hospice, and utilizing art as a medium for healing, began in the 1990s while caring for her dying husband. Today, Robin provides emotional and practical support to hospice patients and their caregivers, assisting them through the very personal and unique journey of death. I was also given helpful input from Sarah Marsh, MDiv, and Janelle Womack, LPC. To my wonderful colleagues in the hospice world and dear friends who have been caregivers: you inspire me. My special love to Flo and Jerry, Jeremy, Terry, Meagan, Felice, Culture Club, and Susan. Great gratitude to Karrie Filios, LPC, for believing in me. Without Chris's writing, this book would never have been born. Thank you for allowing me to be part of Esther's life and yours.

And blessings to the beyond to my cousin Nancy Garment for letting me share your life and death, nephew Danny Buesser and father-in-law Stan Amdurer, Carrie Blankfield for your wisdom, my father, Carl Schlesinger for your perseverance and mom Renée Schlesinger for your devotion. Amen v'amen.

From Chris ...

For unending encouragement and support, for bad jokes and gracious and freely spoken prayers, for running errands, Grandma-sitting, and bringing Ding Dongs, I give profound and endless love and thanks to the innumerable who smoothed the edges of this jagged and relentless journey: my devoted and selfless husband, Kevin; loving and quirky children, Andrew, Cara, Jayme, Will, and Caroline; brilliant and whimsical grandchildren, Colin, Ellie, and Natalie; dutiful and incomparable siblings, Tim, Wendy, Dan, Lexi, Jens, and Steve; dear and abiding nieces and nephews, Mandi, Trenton, Sean, Geli, Kim, Connor, Candi, and Zak; treasured and thoughtful friends and cousins, Pastor Rob, Lee Ann, Melinda, Molly, Lisa, Rodney, Tammy, Jelena, Jean,

Bruce, Moriah, Janet, Steve, Stefanie, Doug, Tres, Denise, Nancy, Patrick, Nate, Nancy, Dena, Dianne, Lynn, Terri, Chuck, Alhana, Jeni, Cheryl, Stacey, Doris Jean, Donnie, Farrell, Nathaniel, and Natalie; my gifted and beloved students; my Facebook community; The Elderly Parent Caregiver Support Group, Dr. Amundson, St. Anthony's Hospice staff, Mary and Stephanie; Lutheran Church of the Master, Rocky Mountain Corvair Society of America, Hostess for making Ding Dongs, Downton Abbey creator, Julian Fellowes, Tia for her mission to comfort the grieving and for her vision for this book and diligence in seeing it through, and above all, Mom and Dad. I miss you.

1

THE MESSY JOURNEY: HOW DID I GET HERE?

On this day, after nearly thirty years of marriage, I learned that my husband really meant it when he said, "for better or for worse."

Just when you thought you were safely through child-rearing and might be looking at some downtime—or time to go back to school or perhaps do some long-awaited traveling—you discover that your family member is not as self-sufficient or healthy as you had hoped and more care is needed. For some, this is an expected journey as a caregiver. For many others, the idea of becoming a primary caregiver means negotiating with siblings, your spouse or immediate family and identifying the financial realities which may drive the type of facility you choose for your loved one.

How can the words caregiver and caretaker mean the same thing? [In this book, we choose to use the term caregiver which feels to us more holistic.] Taking care of someone else is a remarkable thing. You may be looking out for their physical well-being as well as trying to allay their fears and provide nurturing comfort. You may be giving them their medications as well as taking care of the doctor's visits. You may be learning family history that has never been told before or regretting memories that will never be made.

The choice to become a caregiver may be based on cultural expectations. It may be your background in health or elder care that makes you the most suitable for this task. Perhaps you are the one unmarried sibling or the only child so this role falls to you. It may be that your home is big enough to accommodate an extra person. It could be your parent's choice of location. Whatever has brought you to this moment, know the reality of caregiving is so much more complex than can be detailed here. It can fill you with great love and humility and it can bring out incredible pettiness and frustration you never imagined.

To get through this time in a healthy way with self-compassion, you will need support—both physical and emotional. Even the most loving and respectful relationships are tested when roles shift, health declines, and independence wanes. For some, siblings or a partner may be the person(s) to provide hands-on support, but others may need to look beyond the obvious for a village of friends.

I never imagined that one day we would be in our former marital bedroom transferring my mother from her hospital bed onto the bedside commode. Mom's instinct is to flail and grab for anything within her reach, but when my husband says, "I gotcha!" she is reassured and remembers to hold onto him. "I gotcha," is Kevin's way of saying, "Don't worry, I've got your back, I'm supporting you, you're safe." He says, "I gotcha!" and she knows he does. He keeps his eyes focused on the ceiling, and I take care of the dirty work. For better or for worse, "I gotcha!"

For better or for worse, "I gotcha!"

Sometimes when your elderly mother lives with you, you might feel as though you are beginning to lose your fierce sense of independence. To avoid being noticed, you will revert to less than honorable teenage behaviors and start slinking around the house. You might even hide in the basement, pretending you don't hear her when she calls your name.

After she goes to bed, you sneak upstairs to make yourself a cup of peppermint tea. You are careful not to turn on the light, as you know she always sleeps with her door open. You don't want to relinquish this rare moment of mom-free solitude. Without the light, you won't see your black cat, who is lurking about, surveying your late-night activity. You will trip over him, dropping the tea kettle as you turn to place it on the stove. "Shit!" you exclaim, and "Ow!" as you bang your toe against the cabinet. You quickly wipe up the spilled water, but then you hear it: "thump, sniff, scratch, slurp." Your mother is making her way into *the kitchen. Even with her hearing aid out for the night, she still hears you. You panic, grab your phone and leap out of the danger zone. You quickly realize you won't have enough time to retreat to the basement without being seen, so you dive into the coat closet, wedging yourself in between the vacuum and the tripod. Sanctuary!*

It's all your husband's fault, you surmise. You asked him weeks ago to order you an invisibility cloak. "Backorder, my ass!" After all, he is the nerdiest of geeks. He has connections! He knows LARPers! He plays D&D! A standard perk of being married to one of them, one would think. What good is he if he can't acquire an accoutrement as basic and essential as an invisibility cloak???

As you quietly crouch in your dark, yet cozy hideout, waiting for the threat of invasion to pass, you begin texting your children, telling them of your predicament. Your son is surprised there is room enough for you to take refuge in the coat closet. Everyone knows that opening the door to that over-stuffed repository could result in almost certain blanket bombardment or umbrella impalement. Your daughter suggests rifling through coat pockets for snacks and reading material. She's always thinking. She recommends gathering an emergency kit of candy and crosswords for subsequent coat-closet-crisis. "Your new hidey place is already equipped with pillows and blankets," your child points out. You begin making plans to install soundproofing and a mini kitchen. Sure to provide comfort for any future closet-diving situations.

Boredom begins to set in as you wait for the coast to clear. You download a candle app onto your phone to add a little mood lighting to your space. You think you might just nest 'til dawn. And as you sit there in your tight quarters with the faint glow of your iPhone candle, your legs cramping and your feet tingling, you begin to question your morality and hope there will still a place for you in heaven when you someday finish this onerous and capricious journey.

⟋⟍

Building Community

Some may find comfort in a faith tradition and it is always a good thing to ask your religious leader for support. Ask for help when you need it. For many, the greatest stress relief can be found in caregiver support groups, whether in person or online. Many churches and Assisted Living and Memory Care facilities have monthly groups, and the Alzheimer's Association also provides coping groups. Call your local hospice to find other meetings. Get to know your neighbors. Join an exercise class or sign up for an activity you like, just to get out of the house. Stay in touch through social media as you feel comfortable.

Know this can be a marathon and you will need to take breaks from the emotional and physical turmoil. This can be a topsy-turvy time. The parent you respected may be truculent or unable to communicate. You may be performing diaper changes for the parent who did the same for you. There is no one way to manage this, so laugh when you can, share tender moments when possible, and practice self-care.

Finally, remember to reflect on who you are as an individual, and not just the title "caregiver." Some well-meaning friends may compliment your ability to take on this role or note you are providing the best possible care, but these accolades can feel hollow if you feel you have given up a great part of yourself to take on this task. Remind yourself of your multi-faceted personality and tend to the needs of your soul.

The Rest of the Family

Understand that caregiving can trigger all sorts of power struggles, not only with the parent, but also with your immediate family and your family of origin. Obviously, previous grudges and resentments can play into the drama. In most families there are established roles that carry over from childhood, but things become jumbled when one child takes on the mantle of the caregiver. You may find yourself triggered by the lack of appreciation shown by siblings or their complete denial that you are doing the best possible thing for your parent.

You will be triggered by siblings and your parent.

For siblings who wish to help, you will need to draw very clear boundaries as to what "help" looks like. A sibling who "swoops in" for a week and takes over may want to participate and relieve you of stress, but these interludes can cause more aggravation than assistance. How do you handle this?

Make very clear your expectations, but also leave some wiggle room. There may be lines in the sand—mom cannot go out without her oxygen, dad needs his medications dispensed at 1 pm—and it may be that the guest is not able to see the reality of the patient's stamina. Draw up a list of activities or limitations including how far a person can walk comfortably, times for meals, changes in behaviors. Levels of ability may change frequently, so update the list. A visitor may rent a car and plan to use it without realizing the wheelchair can't be accommodated. If you have free passes to favorite locales or handicapped permits that can be shared, make a note of this.

And then there's the real hurt when your parent expresses great joy at the efforts made by the visitor, leaving you wondering what you've been doing all these months ...

Be on the lookout for your own defensive responses to otherwise well-meaning queries. Another family member may begin suggesting new treatments or what they expect is a fresh approach to a nagging issue. Likely, you will have explored many avenues of which other family members have no knowledge, and while their "help" is frustrating, it may be all they can do. One way to divert from a potential outburst is to calmly write down the suggestions and look at and analyze them at a calmer moment.

You will be triggered by siblings and your parent.

⟨⟨⟨⟩⟩⟩

Nothing ...

Sometimes, when your mother's doctor notices she is losing weight, he might suggest you supplement her meals with Nutritional Shakes. Even though they're expensive, you promptly head to the supermarket and purchase all variety of flavors: chocolate, vanilla, strawberry, coffee latte ... You *even buy the blueberry pomegranate flavor for her. Back at home, you proudly present the selection. She chooses chocolate. She draws a quick sip through the straw and rewards your effort with a long, "mmmMMMmmm ... " You are satisfied that you have effectively altered the course of her weight loss and contributed to her essential health and wellness by being an attentive and devoted daughter.*

You spend the next several months buying nutritional shakes every time you go to the grocery store. You notice she always places her lunchtime shake on her walker and wheels it to her room in the afternoon. She wants to drink down every last, delicious drop, you surmise. She even rinses the shake container out in the sink when she has finished drinking down its exquisite creaminess. You figure she is being proactive in preventing garbage odor caused by sour nutritional shake containers, and you are pleasantly surprised by her industriousness.

What you do not know is that your mother really does not like nutritional shakes. You would never have guessed except you enter her room one day at the precise moment she is flushing Butter Pecan down the toilet. You ask her what she is doing, and she quickly turns to see she's been caught. "Nothing," she says. Now, you are a mother, and you've heard this culpable response countless times. Heck, you used that evasive tactic on her more times than either she or you can remember. ... "Chrissy, what are you doing?" "Nothing." (While slipping open the wrapping of one of your Christmas presents.) ... "Chrissy, what are you doing???" "Nothing." (Upon giving both the neighbor kid and his dog haircuts with your mother's sewing scissors.) ... "CHRISSY! WHAT ARE YOU DOING???" "Nothing!" (After sending baby brother, Timmy, down the stairs for a ride in his walker.)

You know when anyone quickly turns and claims, "Nothing," after you ask, "what are you doing," they are guilty of something. How long, you wonder, has she been flushing shakes down the toilet? Why couldn't she just tell you she didn't fancy them? You would have happily searched for something more to her liking. Was this payback for all the times she caught you in a fib as a child? You thought payback was supposed to come in the form of your children misbehaving, not your mother ...

You are responsible for her welfare. You can't let her waste away ... If she loses more weight, you are not adequately doing your job as her caregiver. You can't punish her. You can't force her to eat. She won't tell you what she wants ... Once again, you are defeated. "Chrissy, what are you doing?" "Nothing ... "

NOTES AND THOUGHTS

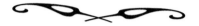

2

THE HARD CONVERSATIONS

...

Dad: "Give me back my license and my car." Me: "Dad, you'll have to be able to lift your oxygen tank and walker into the car to be able to drive." Dad: "Oh, I can do that. Give me my car and my license so I can drive it over a cliff." Me: "You'll have to lift your oxygen tank first, then you can drive anywhere you want."

Stripping away the last vestiges of independence from your aging parent is probably one of life's more difficult tasks. It acknowledges that roles have changed and your loved one now needs to rely on your judgment to keep him or her safe. Some folks have had their parents carefully and neatly moved to a retirement village, independent living or assisted living campus with little drama. In many cases, this first move may be initiated by the parents themselves. But at the time there is a need for a skilled nursing facility, rehab center, or hospice there can be emotional changes that rock the tranquility. Not only are your parents struggling with this transition, you and loved ones are feeling the beginning of anticipatory grief.

While many children are able to work with their parents to go through a lifetime of memories needing to be condensed to a few rooms, often this is a time of high stress for the family. Who gets the family heirloom and what do we do with the china that no one wants? How do you respectfully announce to your father that driving his beloved car is no longer safe? How do you insist to your bookkeeper mother that she can no longer balance her own checkbook? What about that Do Not Resuscitate order?

Some of the things mom packed for dad for his most recent nursing home stay:

- *Nail polish remover*
- *Two nail files*
- *Her left hearing aid*
- *A nearly empty bottle of Old Spice*
- *3 pairs socks*
- *2 pairs underwear*
- *1 pair slacks*
- *1 shirt*

I slipped in a few more socks and underwear and some sweat suits and put the nail polish remover back in the bathroom. I left the hearing aid, nail files, and Old Spice bottle, and moved everything into a small suitcase. I think it was sweet she lent him one of her own hearing aids and that she wanted him to smell good. She was trying to help make his stay more pleasant for both him and the staff!

∽

Start Planning Early

A standard living will is the document approved by an attorney, signed and witnessed, describing your wishes about being kept alive by various means under specific circumstances. You may decide when you wish to be resuscitated or rely on medical interventions, all enforced by a person you designate as your Health Care Proxy or Medical Durable Power of Attorney.

Five Wishes® is published by Aging with Dignity www.agingwithdignity.org. This slim booklet is basically a living will that lets you say how you want to be treated at the end of life. Forty-two states recognize that once signed, this document can supersede a previously filled out advanced directive, living will or durable power of attorney for health care. According to the document, after you sign your *Five Wishes* and follow directions for witnessing or notarizing, to ensure your wishes are followed either destroy old copies of living wills or durable power of attorneys or write "revoked" across your copy.

Five Wishes provides a format that is clear and encourages discussion among family members. Many people have wills that specify their wishes. However, by actively discussing your choices while you are healthy, your loved ones know what you want. If you have questions about this, contact a legal or medical professional in your state. Additional detail can be found in the comprehensive booklet, *Hard Choices for Loving People*, by Hank Dunn (www.HankDunn.com)

Some Terms to Know:

DNR

Do not resuscitate—this means that no medical intervention will be used should your heart stop. If you have doctor-signed DNR form or bracelet as visible proof, emergency personnel will not attempt CPR (cardio-pulmonary resuscitation). Without this indication, they will.

MDPOA

Medical durable power of attorney—the health care agent you have chosen to make decisions on your behalf. Usually, this is a family member, but it does not have to be. There may be a primary MDPOA and others who can take the role if needed. This function ceases at time of death.

POA

Power of attorney—strictly for financial and legal purposes if you are incapacitated; this role ends at the time of death.

Legal Guardian or Conservator

These terms are used when a court has determined that an individual is mentally incapacitated and unable to make decisions on his/her own behalf.

ALF

Assisted Living Facility—the services provided by this type of residence differ from state to state and by management company. Generally, a person living in an ALF is cognizant and may or may not be able to self-administer medications. Hospice care may be available depending on certain circumstances. If you are considering this option know what the limitations of care are and be aware that medical support may be limited.

SNF

Skilled Nursing Facility—residents require a higher level of medical care which can be either short-term or end-of-life. This is a nursing home/center where residents have 24-hour support, including access to nurses, CNAs, social workers, and therapies.

CNA and QMAP

Certified Nursing Assistant/Aide who will provide "cares" for a patient, including bathing, toileting, companioning, feeding, dressing, and possibly other duties that are not medical, although certain states allow CNAs to aid with some medical procedures. In some states in order to dispense medication coursework must be done to function as a QMAP (qualified medication administration person).

ADL

Activities of Daily Living are routine activities that people generally do without needing assistance: personal hygiene, dressing, eating, maintaining continence and transferring (from seated to standing or getting in and out of bed). Instrumental ADLs are more nuanced, such as ability to communicate specific needs. ADLs are considered in determining safety and independence.

POLST

(Physician's Order for Life-Sustaining Treatment) or MOST (Medical Order for Scope of Treatment—Colorado only) forms—a doctor-signed care plan for end of life treatment.

How to Begin the Conversation ...

If at all possible, a discussion around "twilight years" should be held in a neutral setting with limits around the discussion. Plan to introduce the topic of end of life wishes a few days prior to a get together. Share copies of Five Wishes with those who are part of the conversation. Allow for sharing but try to redirect if the discussion becomes heated. It is more than okay for a person to take some time to complete the document. In families where there is a disagreement about end of life care, have one family member represent and rephrase the older adult's comments. For some folks, having a spiritual leader to talk with may be helpful.

When discussing specific restrictions for an older adult, writing down why these actions are being taken may be helpful. For example, when taking a parent's car keys, it can diffuse the anger to have a list of times when he or she got lost while driving, had a fender bender, neglected to repair a headlight, acknowledged feeling scared while on the highway, had vision issues, etc. Stress that this action is to prevent a tragedy that might seriously injure someone else. Additionally, a list of compensatory travel arrangements can help—transport by taxi, car service, private bus, etc.

While many people prefer to age in their home, if the home is unsafe or frequent ER visits are making living at home untenable, moving to a relative's or a group home or retirement village can be an option. Planning for this should take several months just to decide the best option financially and emotionally.

These changes are likely to have an emotional impact on both the parent and the children. Parents may feel they are being forced into decisions they don't like and are afraid of. As the child now taking a caregiving role, you may find resentment, anger or frustrations when your parent continues to berate or blame you. The sadness of giving up a childhood home may impact you in ways you were not prepared for. These emotions can get intense, and it is helpful to begin to find your support system and develop techniques by which you can process these feelings, such as journaling or regular exercise.

In the ER with Mom AND Dad again ... Anyone want to try telling my 88-year-old father that climbing a ladder and having his 87-year-old wife steady it for him is a REALLY BAD IDEA???!!!!

We moved Mom and Dad to an independent living facility today. Leaving them tonight was like leaving Andrew in his dorm room for the first time, leaving Cara after Colin was born, and leaving Jayme on the first day of kindergarten. It never, ever gets easier. Ever.

NOTES AND THOUGHTS

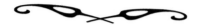

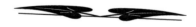

3

WHAT DOES "CAREGIVING" MEAN?

All I want is to walk with her and comfort and care for her on this journey. To be graceful and worthy of grace.

Many folks have a choice in where their loved one spends their final days. There is no shame in choosing a facility that provides activities, nursing care, and entertainment that your family can afford. Residency in group homes or high-rise luxury buildings are possible, as is the aging in place philosophy where help comes into the home round the clock. Many elders enjoy being in an environment where meals and cares are provided by professionals and worries like check-writing or housekeeping are not a concern. Selecting a living facility for your loved one will involve questions around location and price. Safety and continuum of care will be other aspects to consider.

All nursing homes that participate in Medicaid and Medicare are required to be licensed and are rated yearly by a state survey. Before selecting a care facility to visit, check results at Medicare.gov. Ask questions of the facility including worst-case scenarios—what is the protocol if my parent falls? Is there a memory care unit on site? How often will a doctor visit? If my parent needs overnight attention, can someone sleep over?

Get to know the personnel at the facility. If there is a social worker on site, he or she will be the appropriate liaison for making appointments with staff. If there is an activities director, you as a caregiver can assist in providing information about games, music, or field trips that might be of interest to your loved one.

The most demanding, most challenging, most difficult task I will ever undertake is being the kind of daughter my mom needs me to be.

Most people find the responsibility of caregiving greater than they could have imagined. The inability to find time for self-care is a huge problem. Recognize that none of us is super-human and being a caregiver is an emotionally and physically draining job. Ask for help with chores that need doing. Ask for companionship for your loved one, or pay for a companion. Make time for self-care. Join a support group and acknowledge your different feelings about this time.

Being a home caregiver is not a task everyone can do—recognize your family and home limitations. Whether duty, love or financial implications are the driving force, weigh the options and reconcile yourself that you are providing the best care you can. Only you can decide what is possible for your family. And simply because your parent is not under your roof, it does not mean that your responsibilities are less important than those of a child who is able to care for a parent in their own home.

Kevin's Experience: Love Goes in

I asked to be included because, while Chris speaks extraordinarily well for those who are taking care of an elderly parent, there's one highly impacted group of people for whom she can't speak: those of us who live with the person who is taking care of an elderly parent.

When Chris asked if we could move Esther into our home, I immediately said yes. At least I hoped it sounded immediate to her, but I really didn't want to do it. I'm a private person who only finds comfort from the stresses of the world by hiding and recovering in my home. My sanctuary. Adding another adult to my sanctuary just turns it into one more place from where I need to hide. However, in talking to both Chris and Esther, I heard their sincere desire to repair a relationship that, while neither of them openly admitted to each other was strained, both knew it was at best cordial and could—and should—be so much better. They both longed for a strong mother-daughter relationship, and here was their chance. How could I say no to that? And besides, how bad could it be?

Bad. It could be bad. Really, really bad. Every day seemed to get worse. We started out with hope. Chris worked hard to integrate Esther into our routines, but that didn't really work. Looking back, I get it. Esther had many, many years to lock in her routines, and she didn't have the strength or desire to change now. As we gave up on that, Chris decided to at least meet Esther's needs, but that was an elusive target.

As time went on, our home became more and more the main place from where I needed to hide. But where? I hated being at home, but I had nowhere else to go, and even if I did, I would be abandoning Chris, who was suffering so much pain and sadness, and she needed me. I couldn't do that to her. But I found myself living each day with less and less hope and joy. I became withdrawn and surly which added to Chris's stress, which added to my stress, and so on. Our home was not happy.

The hope that they would repair their relationship was long gone. All three of us were just hanging on. I wanted to be a rock for my wife, but I was the wrong kind of rock. Instead of being a strong foundation upon which she could lean, I was just another rock hung around her neck, dragging her down into an abyss of sadness and grief.

Then one day, she showed me an article she found on the Internet which changed my perspective and gave me the ability to be the right kind of rock. In "How not to say the wrong thing,"[1] Susan Silk and Barry Goldman present a simple guide for how to comfort people who are affected by

---

[1] Susan Silk and Barry Goldman. How not to say the wrong thing." Los Angeles Times, April 7, 2013. Accessed November 2, 2017. http://articles.latimes.com/2013/apr/07/opinion/la-oe-0407-silk-ring-theory-20130407

trauma. It starts by drawing a circle and placing the name of the person at the center of the trauma. In our case, it was Esther. Then draw another circle, putting the name or names of those most closely affected. For us, this was Chris. Continue drawing circles and placing names. I came next. The rule with the circles is that the person in the center gets to dump their emotions, fear, grief, anger, etc. outwards, but only comfort goes inwards. If you're angry or afraid, those emotions can go out, but not in. Silk and Goldman state it thusly: Comfort IN, dump OUT.

Support and love go into the circle, and anger and sadness out. Simple. But where was out? Since my life was narrowed to work and home, I began sharing openly and honestly with my friends at work. OK, I really was just complaining bitterly. But as guilty as I felt in dumping my problems on them, I never regretted it. I found great comfort in their kindness and caring, which was made even more powerful because they were supporting me. Only me. Not Chris or Esther. I've always thought of myself as a person with few friends, but I found I was wrong. I have many friends. And now I look for ways to support them as they look out from the centers of their own circles.

We all have a place in the circle. Most of the time it's on the outside, hopefully way, way outside, but for all of us, there will be a time when we get dragged towards the center. Recognizing that sometimes it's just not all about you, even when your entire being is screaming that it IS all about you, will give you the strength and ability to survive. As Esther became more and more ill, and as our world shrank around us, I survived by repeating to myself: Be patient. You can do this. Use the circle. Anger goes out. Love goes in. Love goes in. Love goes in.   —Kevin

Trying to be the best mom for my kids, I thought, was the most demanding job I would ever have. Turns out being the kind of mom my kids needed was a piece of cake. I have great kids. They make everything easier. Then, somehow, I summoned the courage to return to school at age 48. This was the most difficult thing I would ever do. I was sure of it... Nope ... Not even close. It seems the most demanding, most challenging, most difficult task I will ever undertake is being the kind of daughter my mom needs me to be.

We make a good team. Unstoppable, really.

Mom is ever resistant to help, and the day to day, minute to minute challenges are overwhelming. I am beyond blessed to have Kevin treading along beside me, and our kids covering our backs as we sojourn. We make a good team. Unstoppable, really.

"Job" Description

The description of a caregiver's function depends on many variables. If your parent is in a care facility, you may find yourself:

bringing home and laundering dirty clothes, attending functions there, visiting daily/weekly, meeting with the facility staff to discuss behavior changes or concerns, being the go-to person for any needs your loved one has, driving your parent to outside doctor appointments, arranging visits from friends and relatives ... and perhaps holding down a job and maintaining a family home.

If you are an at-home caregiver, some of your responsibilities may include:

adjusting for safety precautions around the home— such as installing grab bars, removing throw rugs and acquiring non-slip mats, having a working fire extinguisher, checking that the water heater thermostat is set below 120°F, preparing for durable medical equipments (such as commodes, hospital beds, oxygen tanks/cylinders), being available to drive to appointments as necessary, providing meals to your loved one that may be different than the norm, monitoring medications ...

If you are preparing your home for an elderly relative, here are some things to consider:

- a phone they can hear on
- a simple-to-use remote
- furniture that can move to accommodate a walker
- ramps
- TV access in the bedroom
- shower seat
- lift chair
- coffeemaker
- bed lamp and night lights
- baby monitor

Trying to stay organized is likely one of the most difficult parts of a caregiver's life. How do you attend a care conference when your boss insists you need to present at a sales meeting at that very time? What are your priorities? How do you juggle everything without losing your sanity?

Getting a white board and large sized paper calendars is helpful as are shared calendars with other family members. While many elders are at ease with digital technology, being able to see appointments written in large print can be comforting particularly when memory begins to go and triple-checking is needed. Create a list of people you can count on for specific chores—and utilize them!

As the roles shift in this new world, look for what others can provide based on their strengths. Can you call upon your brother-in-law to do occasional chores? Can your aunt who lives across country call and chat once a week? Can you accept the services of the neighbor's son to mow the lawn for you? And don't forget that your loved one may have requests that others can fill—for example, your parent may enjoy watching birds outside the window. A friend or neighbor might be tickled to be able to fill the need for a bird feeder.

You know you are a caregiver when the only thing you can manage to plan for Valentine's Day is, ahem, "fooling around" after you send your mother to bed. For the love of God, don't forget to turn off the baby monitor!

I am offering bribes to anyone willing to take my dad to the butt doctor today. Anyone?

4:00 am call to take my dad to the ER. We will be welcoming a new little kidney stone into the family very soon.

ﮩﮩ

One step forward, three steps back ... When your mother ends up in the ER after dislocating her hip during physical therapy. While you are there your father calls an ambulance to bring him to the ER for a bloody nose.

─────ﮩﮩ─────

And What Does Your Loved One Need?

What is the meaning of life? While this question is unlikely to be answered here, it is a critical issue for someone facing the end of life. Have I made a difference? Am I a burden? What will I be remembered for? Can you forgive me for ... ?

Your parent is probably experiencing a huge change in his or her worldview. For those who continued to work late into life, the idea of not being useful or being consulted or even being independent is a vital shift. Take the time to talk with your parent as honestly as possible. Depression among the elderly is prevalent. Look for groups where seniors can gather to share stories and enjoy activities where they have peers around them. For some elderly parents, adult day care centers are an excellent option.

Listen to their concerns about feeling trapped or useless. Recognize their emotions are legitimate and validate them. We cannot usually solve these issues, but acknowledging them is one way to help process what is transpiring. During discussions like this, it can be helpful to draw on their previous interests and adapt these to current circumstances.

One elderly woman who was an artist became a mentor to an adolescent who enjoyed art. Together, they would paint and chat and the pre-teen provided companionship while she gained insight. Designating a friend or relative to help your parent record information in a photo album can create bonds as well as a life record. Making useful compilations of their life's work and collections helps confirm life's purpose.

Especially when the patient is not able to function at the level that they used to, they do not want to be seen as a millstone around their family's neck. It will be up to someone in the family to find tasks and chores that are appropriate and helpful.

Watch out! 88-year-old on a mission! She's carting groceries bag-by-bag on her walker from the front door where Kevin has deposited them to the kitchen. She says she needs more exercise. She likes picking things up and pushing them around on her walker: her coffee cup, lunch, shoes, and a nickel.

NOTES AND THOUGHTS

4

ALZHEIMER'S, DEMENTIA AND PERSONALITY LOSS

FYI: If anyone has an urgent question or comment for the President, Dad's nurse's call button is apparently a direct line.

True story: The dreaded phone call at 3 am. As you jolt yourself from a sound sleep, you try to take a breath, calm your racing heart and grab the phone. "Hello?" "Honey, it's Mom!" "Mom what's wrong, why are you calling?" "I'm so sorry, but you need to help me!" "Of course I will. Are you okay?" "Yes, I'm in my apartment." "Okay, what's the matter?" "I can't find my phone!"

The cruelty of dementia has no bounds. Robbing the family and loved ones of an individual inch by inch before the body has time to react. It is a cruel twist of nature.

Dementia takes many forms. Alzheimer's is a form of dementia that can only truly be diagnosed after death through an autopsy. The brain becomes incapable of functioning until it shuts down. For some, a stroke changes the personality, creating an angry dysfunctional person. Vascular dementia may show up with confusion, language deficits and vision loss. Lewy Body dementia also is characterized by outbursts and aggressive behaviors. For a more detailed understanding of the types of dementia go to the Alzheimer's Association website,[2] the Alzheimer's foundation website,[3] or consult with a geriatrician.

Whatever type of dementia your loved one may be afflicted with, it is so important to remember that you are no longer dealing with the lucid and logical parent who once made clear decisions. No matter how you try, you will be unable to connect the dots that once made sense in their lives. This is often the hardest part for adult children of the aged: accepting that logic is no longer accessible.

Dad called early this morning to tell me he spent the night with three stewardesses in their apartment. Whoa, Dad! A conversation later in the morning revealed he had worked with three different therapists in the physical therapy department. If you need travel arrangements with your medical care, St. Anthony's is the place to go!

That awkward moment when your dad wishes you a "Happy 50th Birthday" while he's sitting on the toilet, and it's not your birthday, and you're not 50.

---

2   www.alz.org
3   www.alzfdn.org

Communication between spouses who are 87 and 88 years old, hard of hearing, and in separate medical facilities:

Dad: "I'm calling you from a cell phone!"
Mom: "What?!"

Dad: "I'm calling you from Chris's cell phone!"
Mom: "Oh! Hehehe. Are you OK?"

Dad: "What?
Mom: "Are you OK?"

Dad: "I got to ride in an ambulance!"
Mom: "What?"

Dad: "How did I get in this bed?"
Mom: "Best wishes."

Dad: "What?"
Mom: "OK, bye."

Dad: "OK, bye."

Resetting What Is "Normal"

As difficult as this is, you cannot:

- make them remember,
- change their new-found beliefs,
- help them reason, or
- provide assurances that relieve their anxiety.

Your job has become to simplify, calm, redirect and comfort. Many elderly with dementia understand in the beginning what is being lost and the frustration and fear is obvious. Acknowledge their pain; recognize the magnitude of their loss and be there to let them know that you will not forget—that you will be their trusted companion, even through the suspicion that follows.

Some form of paranoia is frequent—why did you take my car keys? Who's paying for this apartment? Why can't I have my checkbook? That isn't my signature on that document! Where is my husband—what have you done with him? As heart-breaking as this can be, it remains the job of the caregiver to be patient and calm in the face of the storm.

Stay positive: do not try to correct them. Join them in their world as they simply cannot tell reality from fanciful thinking, dreams or stories they've been told. Asking them to think back as to what they've been told before is embarrassing for them as they likely cannot remember or will refuse to believe this has ever been discussed previously.

Do not condescend—encourage
Do not lecture—reassure
Do not shame—distract
Do not command—ask
Do not reason—divert
—*Anonymous meme*

It may be helpful for caregivers and their loved ones to remember some tips for better communication:

- Memory may be better at certain times of the day; later in the afternoon confusion may increase, a phase called "sundowning"
- Talk about broad topics, not specifics

- Phrase your questions in a way that they don't feel anxious if they don't know the answer
- Don't correct or contradict their memories, even when they are wrong; just join them in their world
- Engage with touch, sight and body language
- Your loved one may not be able to follow stories or movie plots; consider reading simple, shorter stories

For many visitors, the idea of coming to see your loved one can be nerve-wracking—will they know who I am? Quite possibly not. Remind visitors that their presence is enough—recognition is less important than feeling attention and being cared for. One very helpful idea to inspire visitors is to create a picture book to look through with your loved one. This scrapbook can be made of generally familiar photos or drawings that can suggest topics to talk about. It is always a good idea to focus on the here and now, bringing their current perception into the conversation.

When words are difficult, branch out. Music can be soothing or bring joy. Playing music from the loved one's teenage years or liturgical pieces—if that resonates with the elder—is remarkable in its ability to bring recall. Songsheets with the words to childhood favorites can be helpful. Simple card games, simple puzzles, or tactile and repetitive activities can be calming to some. However, if it is not of interest or they protest that the activity is childish, do not force it.

Pets who enjoy cuddling can offer great soothing powers. Enjoying nature or watching birds or fish in an aquarium may be just enough entertainment

Often caregivers who have had troubled relationships with parents have a great desire to make things right at the end or a need to have their loved one acknowledge the care, love, and devotion they are getting. When dementia has set it, the world shrinks and comfort and needs of the patient become more and more the focus. Talk to a therapist or a caregiver's group to process your own feeling of "unfinished business."

It is more than likely your loved one will be unable to acknowledge your efforts in a way that will feel authentic.

———— ഇ ————

Words I never imagined I would hear myself say to my mother:

1. *Oy, your breath! Please go brush your teeth.*
2. *You need to take a shower. You're ripe.*
3. *Candy is not a meal. It is a dessert.*
4. *Chips are not a meal. They are a snack.*
5. *Ice cream is not a meal … Oh, never mind.*
6. *Stop watching me!*
7. *Stop following me!*
8. *If you're bored, go find something to do.*
9. *Say, "Please."*
10. *Say, "Thank you."*
11. *If you can't hear me, TELL me!*

12. *Chrissy put your dress down. (OK, I don't say this one, but it's one she used to say to me, a lot.)*
13. *Spatulas don't go in your underwear drawer.*
14. *The phone won't turn on the TV.*
15. *You can't call Tim on your remote.*
16. *Stop giving me money!*
17. *No, I'm not going to find someone to give your old housecoat to.*
18. *Don't wash your underwear in the toilet.*
19. *I'm not going to save your pizza crusts for lunch tomorrow.*
20. *GO TO YOUR ROOM!!!*
21. *We don't need to save the yogurt cups, frozen food trays, and Gatorade bottles to eat out of.*
22. *Don't put your food down the disposal and tell me you ate it all.*
23. *Use your words.*
24. *Please wear underwear.*
25. *Please say, "Excuse me," instead of running into me with your walker.*
26. *Yes, we have to go to church.*

NOTES AND THOUGHTS

5

ANTICIPATORY GRIEF AND ALL THOSE UGLY EMOTIONS!

"What color were Dad's eyes?" As innocuous as it was as she spoke it, Mom's query caused a ping in my heart that altered its very shape. My soul will forever host the sadness and permanence of her question. How bad had her memory gotten? I tried to picture his eyes in my mind. "Brown," I said. "No, hazel." Were they hazel? Jens's eyes are brown, Danny's are hazel, mine are green, and Mom and Tim's eyes are blue. I'm sure they were hazel ... I think. Why didn't I remember?

For caregivers, the range of emotions that crop up include everything: loneliness, regret, remorse, grief, denial, fear, anger, sadness, pity, gratitude, resentment, happiness, frustration, and more.

There is no right way to feel at this time just as there is no right way to grieve. Because each of us has a complicated relationship with our parents and with our contemporaries, the struggle to stay present is real.

You may be facing the prospect of becoming the elder statesperson in your family. The transition from son or daughter to family patriarch or matriarch is huge. We are reminded each day that life is limited. We may begin contemplating what life will look like down the road. Even when the relationship is not a good, the loss of an adversary still leaves a hole.

*There is no one way
to handle the emotions
that are stirred up.*

Anticipatory grief can be thought of as the mind and heart's way of preparing for the upcoming death. Just as with a death loss, the incremental passing away of your parent's independence and memory and "adulthood" creates waves of sadness and perhaps anger. For many children, seeing their parent suffer from a debilitating illness is horrific and the desire for a speedy death is twinned with guilt. When illness robs us of the connections that have made us family, it is normal to feel frustration and loneliness. And when dementia or a stroke or just pain associated with disease makes your loved one cranky or demanding or without an emotional filter, the sneaky emotion of hatred can be present.

These emotions are simply a reaction to a very stressful and uncertain period.

———✺———

When Regrets Surface

I'm so jealous of all of you who enjoy your parents' company and treasure the time you have with them. When do I get past the, "I can't believe this is my life," regretful, resentful stage? I have never used the "F" word as much as I do since my mother moved in.

———✺———

Forgiveness is a big part of end of life, but it is a myth that all relationships can or should be healed; for some, letting go of the pain may be the best they will be able to do. Whether you are able to forgive past wrongs or understand difficult circumstances that may have come to light, you are suddenly under a compressed time constraint to "get it all resolved before they die!" Whether or not you choose to forgive, if you just start the process of understanding, or you recognize that you don't need or want to forgive, you should be forgiving of yourself.

There is no one way to handle the emotions that are stirred up at the time. For children of alcoholics or those who have grown up with abuse, abandonment or mental illness, there may be a desire to mend the fences and try to be the best caretaker of all time. These children may hope that their parent suddenly recognizes the wrongs they committed and can somehow become the parent they "should have been." There can be tremendous disappointment in this codependent approach and bitterness and frustration appear naturally.

We often see anger come to the surface. Who is your anger directed at? From where does it stem? Was this a parent who hurt you or who did not protect you? Perhaps there are things you wish you could have changed but felt powerless. I encourage you to explore your anger with a counselor to help work through unfinished business.

Many loving children who become caregivers do so out of duty and obligation. When the caregiving drags on and other relationships are strained because of it, resentment grows. Usually, this is paired with guilt for feeling resentment. This situation is common for the sandwich generation—just when they were getting ready to retire and enjoy time for themselves, there is a new and all-encompassing responsibility.

Be gentle with yourself. Talk to a counselor or join a caregiver's group. Volunteer with an endeavor that makes you laugh. You are not alone in these conflicted feelings. Impending death is an uncertain time and we humans tend to like knowing what to expect.

Some ideas to help manage this emotional roller coaster:

- Journal
- Get outside in nature once a day
- Learn some mindfulness exercises that can help keep you calm in the moment
- Prepare a list of funny movies that you can watch to release some emotions
- Listen to a playlist of calming or exuberant songs

I gathered all the color photos I could find, scanned them into my computer, and displayed them on the 52-inch flat screen television in our living room so Mom could view them clearly. We examined each one; zooming in to study his eye color. We smiled at the images but talked little about the memories. Sadly, the pictures weren't vibrant enough to discern his eye color. I'd ask my brothers when I talked to them next, I thought, though I didn't. Mom hadn't brought it up again. It was painful, or it slipped through one of the holes in her memory. So I stored that pain and that memory deep in my own heart for her.

⌒☞⌒

The Quiet Moments

It's the quiet moments that are most difficult. ... Not the times I'm thinking about what to fix for dinner, or if I remembered to give mom her pills, or if my daughter is getting enough sleep with a newborn to care for and a toddler to chase after ... Those are the easy times. Those are the moments my mind is occupied. I am programmed to disallow time for reflection and sadness. No, it's the moments I let my mind settle that are painful.

When I am alone and give myself permission to contemplate. When the grandchildren have gone home, my husband is in our bedroom reading, and my mother is snoring softly in her bed. It is then I release the constant and mundane mental chatter that occupies my daily activity, and I remember my father passed away only a year ago. He was nothing short of "feisty" and I remember the legacy of anger and resentment he left behind.

I think about all my family has given up to bring my mother into our home and how we try to invite her to share the warmth and love that grows here, but she refuses it. She's more comfortable with the former. I wonder if I have done the right thing—moving her in. I realize my limitations ... If only I were more forgiving, more selfless, less stubborn ... if I prayed more ... I know she and I are both secretly, silently waiting for an end ... THE end ... and I hate myself for letting this finality to leak into my thoughts.

I should be grateful for the time we have together. And I should shift my thinking so that all the annoyances are just that: annoyances, endearing. Like the Kleenex, the pieces of tissue I find myself wading through and digging out of the crevices of her chair and her pockets before I do her laundry. I take refuge in a package of Double Stuf Oreos, yet their sweet, creamy crunchiness sickens me and I succumb to the realization that I've gained some weight. I know the extra layer of padding is my security blanket. A veritable force field protecting me from self-inflicted judgment and my mother's silent, bored, sad, passive, angry, stare.

I remember butting heads with her growing up. A lot. No one ever seemed to know or care who I was, what I stood for, what my dreams were. Hell, I didn't even know. I just knew my vision would not conform to my family's expectation of me. Thirty years finding myself with the help of my husband and my children defined me. I wear my heart on my sleeve, yet my mother still sees me as the person she perceived me to be back then. Every day is a struggle. A battle to uphold my truth and enfold her in it. Her perception constantly tries to pull me in, smother me, and swallow me up.

I overhear the telephone conversations she has with my siblings. Conversations filled with "How are yous, and have nice days, and I love yous." Never does she afford me the same tenderness and affection. In her mind, I have *become my father—the angry, smart-mouthed enforcer. My only consolation is knowing I am doing what my heart tells me is right and good, and my steadfast dedication to my children. I pray they will always feel my love and respect for them. And I pray I will always remember to thank them for their efforts and shower them richly with love.*

NOTES AND THOUGHTS

6

HOSPICE

Mom: "I don't want to go to the Doctor today, I don't feel good."

Me: "That's WHY you go to the Doctor, Mom."

One of the biggest misconceptions about hospice is that it indicates you are at death's door. Current regulations call for hospice to be available for anyone who has a diagnosis of up to six months to live. Often, once hospice has regulated medications and provided structure and care, the patient may become more comfortable and better able to enjoy the time left. The patient will not be able to access curative or life-prolonging medical procedures while on hospice but can take medications to enhance his or her quality of life. Thus, while chemo would not be allowed, oxygen would. Hospice is a Medicare part A benefit but the VA benefit can be used, Medicaid is an option, as well as private insurance. Generally, the cost of all medication and cares associated with the terminal illness is covered as long as it is for comfort and not cure.

Hospice can be accessed either at your place of residence (home, skilled nursing facility, memory care unit, assisted living or independent living facility) or at an on-site hospice. Medicare does not cover room and board for these locations. In too many cases, the patient could have been made comfortable sooner, but aggressive treatment was being continued for no logical reason. This is where it is critical to have the patient's wishes noted prior to serious illness; how much discomfort is reasonable versus the length of days. The hospice intake and admission professionals can help a family make decisions about the best possible choices for the patient.

We found out Tuesday, after a late night trip to the ER that my mom has enlarged lymph nodes in her abdomen, which is most likely a result of Lymphoma. Mom and her doctor have decided she is too frail for surgery, radiation, chemotherapy, or even a biopsy. Because she won't be having a biopsy, we won't know how aggressive the cancer is. We are in a "wait and watch" kind of holding pattern.

We met with a lovely hospice nurse this morning and are confident the hospice team will help keep her comfortable. Currently, she is still getting up, showering, dressing, walking, and eating on her own. She is resting a lot, and not eating much, but not in much pain.

Living Until the End

Father Paul von Lobkowitz, a nurse, monk and one of the first hospice directors in the US once told me, "Hospice is about living until the end." The philosophy of the hospice movement has always been about finding the best way to live as fully as possible in the time allotted us—whatever that means to the patient. Hospice care focuses on comfort and quality of life, but not cure. Hospice is a philosophy of care, not a location.

Hospice can work alongside a facility staff providing additional nursing, CNA, social work and spiritual care support. When a family has an initial care conference with the hospice team and the facility team details are ironed out as to who will be responsible for what areas of care. The hospice team will know that different facilities have different protocols regarding medications and certain locations may have requirements for transport to a hospital even when the patient is on hospice.

The hospice nurse is generally the professional who visits and assesses the patient's condition, reporting back to a medical director/physician and getting updated medication approval. Families are encouraged to call the hospice nurse (often called a Registered Nurse Case Manager) when there is a change of condition: increased pain, new or worsening symptoms, nausea or vomiting, a decrease in urine output, increased restlessness, trouble swallowing or difficulty breathing. Most importantly, you should develop a relationship with the RN case manager and social worker to share your concerns or ask questions.

A general outline of nursing support can include 24-hour on-call access, one to two visits per week, symptom/ pain/medication management, communication with the family, patient, caregiver on health care instructions, a care plan to address patient's care. Note that if your family chooses a hospice, you should receive a patient handbook which lists what you can expect from each member of the team.

When the family is caring for the patient at home, they are given education on how to administer medications as needed and should have a nurse available by phone 24/7. Family members' level of comfort with "personal cares" will be important if you are at home. If, as a caregiver, you feel unable to deal with the intensity of biological changes as your loved one deteriorates, look into hiring a professional to supplement what you do.

Things are getting serious. I think she suffered a stroke. She is weak, she is confused, she can't walk ... she can't even sit up on her own. I am afraid to go to sleep at night, and I am afraid to go into her room in the morning. I am acutely aware of every sound she makes. I am realizing how profoundly ill-equipped and unprepared I am to do what I have to do.

For those of you who receive Hospice care for your parent, what do you have the CNA do? Ours finally started. Mom has been pretty self-sufficient until just recently. I had our sweet CNA help Mom with a shower and brush her teeth. Mary (the CNA) then helped her comb her hair, massaged her legs with lotion, changed the sheets, played with the cat, visited with us, made an order for barrier cream, pull-ups, bed protectors, and an emesis basin, then asked for more to do. I didn't even know that pull-ups were included with hospice care! What else am I missing????

——————

Everything has been a struggle. Still, it seemed the right thing to do to encourage normalcy.

——————

Hospice Team Members

Families who use hospice may find themselves becoming very close to the hospice team. This is as it should be. Hiring professionals who truly care about the patient and the family give a level of comfort found nowhere else in this process. If you are using a hospice, take advantage of the well-trained staff—ask questions of the nurse case manager, speak with the spiritual care coordinator (chaplain), get suggestions and utilize the emotional support from the social worker. Your confidence in caring for your loved one will grow.

Besides the medical director and Registered Nurse Case Manager, there are other important team members. The CNA should be on a schedule to suit your loved one's needs for bathing and other personal cares. The number of visits a week varies depending on the hospice. Because of their role in performing hands-on tasks and comforting the patient, your CNA may become very close to your family and the patient. These trained aides also grieve when their patients die and a good hospice will provide compassionate team care for them.

―――――◦∞◦―――――

"I Think I'm Getting Better"

Over the last month, Mom would say these words to everyone who asked her how she was feeling; the hospice team, the doctor, visitors, and me, even. It always stopped me in my tracks. I was never sure how to respond when she made this claim. Had she forgotten why we have the hospice team coming several times a week to help her? Did she not notice her steady decline? Was she in denial? Was she putting on a brave face, convincing herself she truly was getting better? Was it a habitual response, with no real meaning behind it or was it simply due to her need to tell everyone what she thinks they want to hear?

It seemed cruel to remind her she had untreatable cancer. I chose to respond with, "That's great!" and continued trying to convince her to do the things that made her feel better; eating, drinking, taking her medicine, showering, brushing her teeth, changing her clothes, allowing me to change her sheets and open the bedroom window and curtains to let some fresh air and sunshine in, practicing yoga, playing with her great-grandchildren, accepting visitors, watching Downton Abbey ... Everything has been a struggle. Still, it seemed the right thing to do to encourage normalcy.

―――――◦∞◦―――――

Social Services Support

Medical social workers are trained to offer resources and referrals to the patient and the family in order to cope with the illness and end-of-life care. They have training in providing psychosocial support as well as guiding families through documentation such as advance directives, Medicare, Medicaid, transfers to different facilities, insurances, funeral planning and respite care. It is on the recommendation of the social worker that a trained companion/volunteer from the hospice might be provided, if available.

Spiritual Care Coordinators or Chaplains are professionally trained to provide support both to the religious and non-religious patient. They are there to listen without judgment, offer comfort, help process the emotional stress, converse on issues of faith, have discussions about the meaning of life and death, read or pray in conjunction with whichever espoused faith, and arrange for specific spiritual leaders as requested. Most spiritual care coordinators will have a Masters degree in Divinity and will have completed educational training at a medical facility.

Volunteers may be able to provide respite in the home for a few hours, may read or play card games with the patient, or may offer individual talents such as music, massage or Reiki energy work (providing they are trained and certified by the hospice). Not every hospice has available volunteers, but you should certainly ask if you might be interested.

Visits from trained therapy animals can be arranged through professional organizations and may be a huge comfort.

Finally, hospices are required to provide bereavement services to the family after the death, and when appropriate, anticipatory grief counseling for families who need this. Bereavement may involve phone calls, one-on-one counseling, letters, group meetings and joint memorial services for hospice families. Each hospice will provide different types of bereavement services.

"I Feel Okay"

Yesterday Mom fell. She woke up very weak, dizzy, scared and confused, which resulted in her passing out while using the bathroom. She only suffered a bump on her noggin, thankfully, but I fear we have entered into a new normal. "I feel okay," is her response of choice, now. Mary, Mom's CNA, a gentle, beautiful, sweet angel, has heavenly powers. I'm convinced. Mom is stubborn, proud, and quite passive, but will allow Mary to do the things that she simply refuses to let me do. I think Mary doesn't give her the choice, really.

Mary is here for one hour, five days a week. For one hour, five days a week, Mom allows herself to be helped. For one hour, five days a week, Mom allows herself to be pampered. For one hour, five days a week, I don't have to beg, plead, cajole, or try to read her mind. For one hour, five days a week, I am resigned. I know Mary's magic touch is the best thing for Mom and for me, but I feel like a failure. I want to be the caregiver. I am the child of a Watt and a Renaud—a combination of stubbornness, passiveness, and pride, (and long legs, a high forehead, and sticky-out ears. My dad used to say that his brother, my uncle Hod, had ears that, "looked like a zone cab with the doors hanging open.")

Mom refuses to ask for help, I refuse to read her mind. Still, I don't give up. I can't be Mary, though every day I try. I am the child of a Watt and a Renaud. For thirty years I have worked at channeling my stubbornness into tenacity, my passiveness into patience, and my pride into self-reliance. I have discovered that thirty years is not enough time to separate myself from the attributes my parents gifted me, so I am grateful for Mary, who for one hour, five days a week, succeeds where I fail.

Levels of Care

In rare cases, the patient experiences a period where their illness is no longer progressing as predicted. Hospice regulations require regular evaluations to determine if the diagnosed terminal illness is continuing as might be expected. If the patient's health improves or shows no decline for a period of time, the patient may "graduate" from hospice care. Should this occur, understand that those hospice patients who have been discharged from hospice care may come back on service whenever their disease process again indicates six months of life remaining. Additionally, should specific circumstances require an emergency hospital visit (unrelated to the course of the illness, such as a fall requiring stitches) the hospice team will likely discharge the patient (technically, the patient will revoke services) for the duration of the emergency care, to be readmitted when they return to their residence. This is a Medicare issue to avoid double-billing.

Hospice care includes different levels. Routine care is the norm. Depending on the hospice you have selected, CNAs may be available several times a week or daily. Continuous care refers to skilled nursing care provided for a set number of hours per day for a short time. GIP or general inpatient care is for a short-term stay where 24-hour nursing care is available and needed to manage symptoms. Finally, respite is a short-term stay at a facility for up to 5 days when the usual caregivers require a break from full-time caregiving.

What options are available under hospice? "Comfort measures" are the key. Pain management, the offering of food, fluids, oxygen, massage, personal cares, and companionship or spiritual camaraderie are all covered. People on hospice can go out, enjoy activities where appropriate for their condition, spend as much time as possible doing the things they enjoy. None of the interventions are curative; unnecessary tests and treatments are not part of a hospice plan.

Colin was a little afraid of Grandma sick in her bed, so we assured him that Grandma still loves him so, so much, and she can still play with him. We talked about how he can help her by bringing her snacks and saying, "Hey, Grandma! Do you want to play with me?" So he went straight to the hungry cupboard and picked out snacks for the both of them. Twinkie for Grandma and Rice Krispie Treat for Colin. She ate.

Food and Drink

As hospice patients decline, they begin to need less and less nutrition. Patients may feel full after a few bites. It is an important step for the caregiver to realize that forcing more food on them is not helpful. The rejection of food is a symptom of the illness—bodily systems are not working well and are slowing down. Additionally, for those struggling with a life-limiting illness food can lose its appeal and taste. There may be difficulty chewing, swallowing, digesting and eliminating food. Force feeding may cause choking, vomiting or may result in aspiration pneumonia.

Forcing more food on them is not helpful.

Many caregivers report that small meals including comfort food are helpful. Avoid strong-smelling foods. Offer liquids at the end of meals to avoid filling them up before nutritional food is offered.

One question that is often asked is about IV fluids. Towards the end of life, when normal body functions are not working well, introducing IV fluids can increase the likelihood of shortness of breath, fluid in the lungs, nausea, and edema (swelling) in the extremities. If the patient has a dry mouth, caregivers will be encouraged to use a swab/sponge to provide moistening to the mouth and lips.

After two days of relative energy this week, Mom has hit a wall. Not only energy-wise but also in communication and spirit. It is becoming increasingly difficult for me to guess what she wants and encourage her to be present. Our remarkably patient hospice nurse tried to help by explaining to her she does not have to suffer needlessly from hunger, thirst, boredom, or pain. Mom only responded with, "I know, I know ... " We have begun the monumental task of looking through her photos and having her tell me who folks are. With the help of Jeni and Stefanie, we are scanning and loading the photos into our screensaver. Mom seemed engaged and even lasted longer than her usual 10 minutes. She did make the remark, though, that she would continue her job tomorrow if she's still here.

NOTES AND THOUGHTS

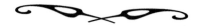

7

CARE FOR THE CAREGIVER

There's a point at which you no longer care about, "Enjoying your mother while she is still here." You just want her to go away.

Self-care is not an ugly word. One of the most exhausting things a person can do is be a caregiver. It requires an enormous expenditure of energy. You may find yourself running ragged on little sleep, having explosive bursts of emotion, worrying about all sorts of details, and trying to manage a household or a job. Your body is practically existing on adrenaline. While going away for a day or two to recharge is not possible for everyone, you should incorporate good self-care into your routine.

Fifteen minute walks daily are a good start. Journal. Color. Take the time to have a nice dinner out; spend an afternoon at a museum or the movies; go shopping for something you want; or go to the gym. Make a habit of this. Being a caregiver can be a long, long journey. Call friends for respite. Involve your faith community or civic group to help you. If hospice is involved, ask for a trained volunteer who can provide companionship or spell the family for time away from the home. This truly takes a village.

Some of you have been asking for specific ways you can help. I am grateful for any and all help! It's true I am a "Type A" personality, and I prefer to keep busy, but I fear I am doing more than any one person should be doing. Accepting your help will keep me in check!

1. *Prayers.*
2. *Short visits with Mom: 30-45 minutes—tops, or by Phone, Skype, or Facetime.*
3. *Run errands. (Or come sit with Mom so I can run errands.)*
4. *Meals. (I hesitate with this one, because of my husband's strange dietary needs.)*
5. *Scanning Mom's photos onto my hard drive so she can easily see them on the screen saver.*
6. *Put Mom's mother's teacups in the special curio cabinet she bought for them.*
7. *Hang a couple of Mom's paintings in her room.*
8. *Find someone with a Chevy Corvair for Mom to take a short ride in. (Her favorite car.)*
9. *Help with Colin and Ellie on the mornings they are here.*
10. *Help taking down my Christmas decor!*
11. *Support for Kevin. He is quiet and unassuming, but surviving minute by minute, just as I am.*

12. Support for my brothers. We are all on different paths of the same journey.

⸺⸱∞⸱⸺

Going away may seem the most callous thing you can do at the end of life. "What if he dies while I'm not there?" Self-care is a truly necessary element, and for long-time or exhausted caregivers, a few days' break can make a huge difference. The patient can be admitted to a care center where their needs are met. Meanwhile, the caregivers get a chance to remember who they are as individuals.

For some families, respite will mean that your loved one will spend several days in a skilled nursing facility while you recoup your own strength. For those on hospice care, this benefit is covered and the hospice social worker should be able to arrange the specifics. The type of respite care ensures that your loved one has attendants available throughout the night and day.

And what about your loved one dying while you are gone? There are two scenarios: one, the patient dies while you are present, and two, the patient dies when you are not. Since this is likely out of the control of the caregiver, doesn't it make sense to take the opportunity to recharge and rest when possible? (More about this in the End of Life chapter.) For those whose parent is on hospice, should a change happen quickly many hospices offer an Eleventh Hour or Transition Team program, where volunteers may sit with your loved one in the event that death is imminent. In any case, whenever there is a significant change of condition or a hospice professional makes an assessment that death is nearing, the next of kin will be contacted as per the plan of care.

⸺⸱∞⸱⸺

Kevin and I are trying to take a little break from everything for a few days. Mom is in respite, Cara has Nick watching the grandkids, and we are driving up to Glenwood Springs to enjoy a concert and stay in a hotel. It's going to be difficult for me to trust that Mom's needs will be met. She will most definitely try to get out of eating and bathing. She'll probably just sit in silence while she's there. I've asked for the boys and grandkids to call ... She will even have visits from our hospice team.

I think my biggest hurdle, though, will be simply switching from "caregiver" to "wife." My days are filled with innumerable caregiving tasks, and I scarcely know who I am if not catering to someone. I have agreed not to call her, per the advice of our hospice team, but I doubt I will comply. I can't abandon her completely. She was very confused about the whole process of being transported and admitted into the respite facility. She thinks she will be living (and dying) there, and doesn't seem to understand that she will be coming back home.

I packed everything she might need for the next few days, including her favorite shampoo and body wash, new magazines, iPad loaded with Downton Abbey episodes and Solitaire, coloring book, extra loungewear and new slippers. The nurses commented that I was, "Such a good daughter," but mom was very clearly in disagreement. Leaving her was not unlike leaving my children when they were young (which was rare). Nonetheless, I will try to enjoy my care "free" time with my husband, and try to remember who I am for a short while.

...My dear snowbound friends, While Mom is relaxing in respite care Kevin and I are getting a few days away. We feel terrible that you all are snowed-in, breaking your *backs shoveling, and suffering from no power while we enjoy 40°F temperatures with no snow, and leisurely strolls through Glenwood Springs shopping and eating. We wish we were there weathering the storm with you, but someone has got to contribute to the Glenwood economy ... If I-70 opens, we will be home tomorrow and can join you in frostbite solidarity then. Thank heavens for awesome neighbors, Kurt and Cheryl who came to Loki, the cat's rescue and fed him!*

<hr />

Henry Ward Beecher said, "Mirth is God's best medicine." During prolonged times of stress, it can be restorative to let go by disengaging from the seriousness of the moment through humor. Recently, health benefits of the simple act of laughing are being researched. According to Sally Abrahms, writing for AARP, laughter yoga was developed in 1995 by Madan Kataria, MD, based on the concept that you get more oxygen to the body while laughing, providing greater energy but also boosting relaxation[4].

Whether by watching funny movies or sitcoms or just listening to jokes, laughter can supposedly relieve pain, lower blood pressure and glucose levels. For the caregiver and support team, finding ways to find humor in a difficult situation may be the break that is needed.

<hr />

4   Abrahms, Sally "Laughter Yoga to Improve Health? It's No Joke." AARP.org. https://www.aarp.org/health/alternative-medicine/info-11-2008/laughter_yoga_to_improve.html (accessed December 8, 2017).

You tell yourself she's not rejecting you ... But you don't believe it.

You can't remember who you are anymore. You have tried, and tried, and tried to engage her, but she is an unwilling participant. Will you feel guilty about not appreciating your time with her? Utterly. Completely. But you need to survive. You have to make it through today. And tomorrow. You tell yourself she's not rejecting you ... But you don't believe it. You are beaten down. Defeated.

Day-by-day, minute-by-minute, you fight your reactions to her dysfunctional behavior. You instinctively respond as her child—ignorant and trusting. But the adult you—fully aware—understands how one should respond. You are not being true to the person you subscribe to be. You try to justify each reactionary decision. You are uniquely gifted in dealing with difficult people. You are perceptive, patient, and empathetic, yet you cannot use those gifts with your mother. Something inside you blocks these traits and forces you to respond as a disconnected stranger. She is eighty-nine years old. She knows no other way. You are the one who needs to change. You know who you are. You've always known, even though she doesn't.

Anyone Hear a Good Joke Lately?

In high school, whenever I was having a bad day, my friend Lisa would always ask me if I wanted to hear a joke. While a joke didn't solve whatever my perceived problem was, when my sweet friend tried to help me feel better with her kindness and humor, it always made me smile. Even if the joke was particularly bad! I am a terrible joke teller, but I learned from Lisa how important it is to see the humor in things.

So ... anyone have a joke to tell??? Lisa???

Rodney: Why didn't the toilet paper cross the road?—It got stuck in a crack.
Chris: Hahahahah! Bathroom humor. Always funny.

Sara: Never tell puns to kleptomaniacs—they always take things literally.
Chris: Good!

Lisa: Knock knock
Chris: Who's there?
Lisa: Euripides.
Chris: Euripides who?
Lisa: Don't bend over or you'll Euripides pants!
Lisa: How's that for a bad joke? Xoxoxoxoxo
Chris: You've still got it! Woot!

Roger: Horse walks into a bar the bartender says, "Hey, why the long face?"

Michelle: What do you call a cow that just had a baby? Decalfinated!
Chris: Hahaha!

Tammy: How do you make a bandstand? Take away their chairs.
Chris: Oh yes! Ha ha ha!

Michele: Knock knock
Chris: Who's there?
Michele: HIPAA
Chris: HIPAA who?
Michele: Can't tell you!
Chris: Groan!!! (Nurses!)

Rick: What is the difference between a fish and a piano?
Rick: You can't tuna fish!
Chris: Chuckle!

Jeni: Why do scuba divers fall backwards off the boat?
Jeni:. Because if they fell forward, they'd still be in the boat.
Chris: Snort!

Cara: Where does the general keep his armies?
Cara: in his sleevies!!!
Chris: Tee hee hee.

Tim : Two blondes walked into a building ...
Tim : You'd think one of them would've seen it.
Chris: Bahahaw!

Chris: Past, Present, and Future walk into a bar. It was tense.

Roger: E-flat walks into a bar, The bartender says, sorry, we don't serve minors ...

Marilyn: I read a review about that new restaurant on the moon. Apparently, it has good food, but no atmosphere.
Chris: Tee hee hee.

Stacey: Why didn't the skeleton cross the road? He didn't have the guts!
Chris: Har har!

Theresa: What do you know if you find bones on the moon?
Theresa: ...the cow didn't make it.
Chris: Groan!

Stacey: Knock knock. Who's there? Dishes. Dishes who? Dishes a bad joke!
Chris: You did good Stacey! Thank you!!! You rock!

NOTES AND THOUGHTS

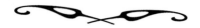

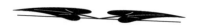

8

BLESSED MOMENTS

Haiku (Sleep)
Invites comfort, soft and warm,
Protector through night's slumber.
Dreams. Healer. Renewed.

A blessed moment is whenever you find it. It can be as simple as enjoying a childhood food, sharing a joke, making a new memory, taking a pause to notice a peaceful or loving interaction. It may be a day when your loved one is awake and cognizant. As a caregiver, these are the things that will stay with you, so be on the lookout for them.

Do not be afraid of laughter with the terminally ill. Should it be your family's temperament to crack jokes and share funny stories at the bedside, do so. Keep in mind that at the end of life, the focus in the room should be on the patient and remember that for those who are not conscious, the last sense to go is hearing—stories and discussion should be appropriate for them. Unless your loved one is asking to discuss final arrangements, keep those conversations out of the room.

Additionally, sharing space or holding a hand or gently massaging a loved one's feet may provide great connection. On one of the last days I spent with my mom, I had the privilege of rubbing cream into her dry, swollen legs which gave her comfort. It was such a small gesture for me, but so appreciated by her.

———⊰⊱———

Sometimes when you have a difficult road to travel, if you're smart, you'll stop and ask for help and direction. When we began this journey through Lymphoma, (and I say "we" because I feel I am traveling this journey with Mom as her "sherpa,") I knew that I could not carry her burden alone. I asked for help, and I asked for direction. Mom and I have received guidance, comfort, and help beyond measure. From my husband who listens to my every gripe and dries every tear, to the daily prayers that are lifted up on our behalf. We are blessed. You all are the calm in the midst of our chaos.

If you're smart, you'll stop and ask for help and direction.

I had asked previously if anyone had or knew of someone who could get their hands on a Chevy Corvair for Mom to take a ride in, to no avail. This morning, with hope, I reached out to the Rocky Mountain Chapter of the Corvair Society of America. Within minutes I received a call from Steve, one of the members who had read my inquiry.

He sounded like Jimmy Stewart, so I liked him immediately, and we chatted at length about Lakewood, Lymphoma, and Corvairs. Steve made it his mission to find a Corvair that was the same year and color of the car Mom owned, or close to it. By early evening he had acquired an early '60's model, baby blue convertible in Castle Rock, owned by a woman who shares my first name, and granted our request with an emphatic, "YES!" Next Sunday afternoon, weather permitting, Steve and Chris will meet us here, take us to Magill's for ice cream, and on a short trek through the Foothills. Mom giggled when she found out. I can't wait to share the pictures.

From the Pikes Peak Corvair Club Newsletter ...

During a February meeting of the Rocky Mountain Corsa Club, a number of members jumped at the chance to give Esther a Valentine's Day gift. A gaggle of Corvairs showed up at the family's cul de sac and Esther was able to choose to ride in a 1960 model. According to the driver, Ed, Esther seemed to be having a great time, chatted about her years teaching in Denver and the various cars the family had owned, including a Model T. Esther shared that the sound and the smell of the Corvair engine was a fond memory! After a visit to the local ice cream shop, the club members made a trip up to the Red Rocks Park in Morrison to enjoy the view and the winding roads.

"Dear Steve and Ed, and Christine, John and Kathy,

Thank you all for giving us such a wonderful experience on Sunday! You are wonderful, selfless, amazing individuals. We were so blessed to have been able to share these moments with you. You made my Mom so happy ... You gave her a little respite from her pain, and we are ever grateful. You also helped her reminisce about some times when her children were little, and life was a little simpler. You gave the rest of us long-lasting memories that we will carry with us always. You have done a wonderful thing.

Sincerely,

Chris Renaud-Cogswell and the Renaud family"

Sharing Stories

Grief counselors, social workers, and spiritual care coordinators encourage the dying and their families to share moments of connection where the patient can recount his or her life's accomplishments. Dying can be hard work psychologically and the patient may need to come to terms with fears and the end of his life here. Having loved ones listen without judgment as the elder examines the meaning of life is a caring gift.

Making and recalling memories is probably the best activity you can engage in at this time. While some folks at the end of life are completely cognizant and able to get around, others may be very weak and unable to expend energy on much beyond conversation.

Your loved one's ability to recall or converse may be limited, but for those who have family or the assistance of the patient, you might consider these prompts to open the door to conversations that are meaningful and memorable.

A few questions at a time is a good rule, with a notebook to take down the answers.

- Where was your family from originally? Did they share things from a particular country, culture or region?
- What are some of your favorite songs?
- What are you most proud of in your life?
- What is your favorite place on earth and why?
- How would you describe yourself? Are there certain times you felt you showed some of your strongest qualities to the world?
- Who was your best friend growing up and what did you like to do together?
- What person influenced you the most?
- What was your first car?
- What Olympic sport would you have liked to try?
- What was the best meal ever? What is your idea of comfort food?
- Are there family stories you'd like to share?
- What would you like to be remembered for?

Veterans and Those with Troubled Pasts

For families whose loved one is struggling with the coming death, educator Deborah Grassman, APRN, says, "Listen, don't corrupt with words." There are times when the patient is resisting death because they are struggling with something weighing on their heart. Sometimes a pastor or spiritual care coordinator is able to hear the painful admissions. Other times, it becomes the family who will help ease the passage simply by listening. Even if the deeds seem shocking, you can acknowledge the courage it took to voice these wrongs and just be present. Ms. Grassman has shared publicly her experience with a dying veteran who confessed to killing many men during war and this responsibility weighed on his soul. Being able to release his life-long shame around this allowed the soldier to let go.

Although the concept of letting go of a parent from this world by "giving them permission to die" and assuring them that you will be okay has become standard, you may find it more appropriate to share music they enjoyed or just recount good times with them. For those whose pasts are troubled—or where the past is unknown—providing companionship on this journey may be all that you can do. Some who are in the process of dying find comfort in meeting with clergy, being anointed, hearing a blessing, or participating in a cultural ritual that releases them.

Memories

October 25

Mom and I got our hair done. This is my first time getting highlights. She can't stop laughing at me. She even twisted my nose to "change the channel". Oh, mom ...

April 19

We found the lamb cake mold mom's Grandma Nielsen gave to her mother; my Grandma Watt. Mom used to make a lamb cake for us every year at Easter, so we decided to make one.

～

November 16

Mom, dusting her harp. It sounds rather like a symphony as she pulls the duster across the strings and adds her own percussive toots when she bends over. I'm calling it the "Elder Harp and Tooter Jamboree!"

～

March 10

After enjoying hotdogs with ketchup with Colin, Mom is resting to Vladimir Horowitz playing Beethoven's Piano Sonata #14 In C Sharp Minor, Op. 27 No. 2 (Moonlight Sonata). I remember her playing it on her baby grand.

～

January 24

Today Mom received calls from her dear friend Betty, and niece Natalie. Per Natalie's genius suggestion, we made æbleskivers for dinner—a traditional Danish food. (Pancakes cooked in a special pan that allows the batter to puff up into balls.)

We tucked fresh fruit inside each one. It was nice hearing her reminisce, and she proclaimed, "You don't eat them with a fork, you eat them with your fingers!" Some things, like cooking one of her favorite childhood dishes, a woman never forgets.

We used Natalie's recipe, and read it straight from her comment to my post from my laptop right on the counter—Mom was gobsmacked! The recipe turned out dozens of perfect fruit-filled pancake puffs.

I Am Grateful For:

- *Tradition.*
- *Long distance calls from dear friends and family.*
- *Memories.*
- *Selfless strangers*

NOTES AND THOUGHTS

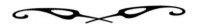

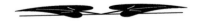

9

END OF LIFE

Mom isn't speaking much, but she is content listening. Jens calls often and talks about memories as she listens. She likes hearing his voice. I think it brings her comfort. She tells him she loves him very much, and that a person should say it very often.

One of the most mystical and reverent experiences can be the end of life. Many professionals liken these moments to birth—the journey from a safe haven to the unknown. But the actual understanding of the event will remain a mystery. Most people state they would like to just die in their sleep, and while this is a real possibility, for caregivers there will be indications that death is nearing.

Watching this process is hard when your role has been keeping your loved one safe and comfortable. Fear of "doing the wrong thing" or wondering "is this normal?" are common themes. Recognizing the signs of impending death may help prepare you to let go.

If your loved one is on hospice, certain medications may be offered to keep the patient comfortable and manage the symptoms associated with his or her illness. Some patients may require anti-psychotics if they are prone to vivid hallucinations. Certain patients may need anti-nausea medications or may be given a drug to inhibit secretions. Folks who are in pain or having trouble with shortness of breath may be offered morphine. These medications are not intended to hasten death, just allow the process to progress easier.

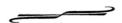

Chris: *"Mom, are you uncomfortable? Do you want some Morphine?"*

Mom: *"I don't want to get addicted to that stuff."*

Physical Changes

As the individual comes to terms with the dying process, they may begin to withdraw and sleep more. Food becomes less important and your loved one no longer enjoys the taste of food. For the family, this change can be very hard to accept because it acknowledges that the body is not being sustained and death is coming. Family members may feel that the rejection of food is a rejection of them. Try to remember that the body is preparing for its final journey.

As death comes nearer, the person may want no fluids and the body experiences dehydration, but without the side effects of a healthy individual. It is appropriate to withhold artificial hydration such as IV fluids eliminating unnecessary edema, and the need for a catheter, urinal or bedpan and to allow the body to reach a state of lessening awareness. For many family members, the use of sponges to keep the mouth and lips moistened is a caring gesture at this time.

Ironically, some folks rally at this stage, gathering energy they have not demonstrated in weeks, and appearing very alert while sitting and talking. Others may gather their belongings as if ready for a journey.

Falls

Another aspect of the physicality of dying that may cause additional concern is falling. Whether due to weakness or lack of balance or trying to pick things up from the floor, a common occurrence is a fall. Even with the most vigilant oversight, patients can tip from a wheelchair or roll out of bed as well. Current regulations have deemed it inappropriate to restrain our elders by tying them into a chair or using bedrails within care facilities. Discuss options like lowering the bed position or utilizing a deep recliner.

Falls may result in an injury that could require medical attention. If your loved one is at home on hospice, discuss with the team in what circumstances it is appropriate to bring your parent to an emergency facility. All falls—even without obvious injury—should be reported to the care team.

⌇⌇⌇

Mom has begun hallucinating. Today she woke up from a nap trying to get out of bed and telling me she can't move. She thought Dad was sitting in his chair in her room. Mom told me he had asked her to pick something up, but she couldn't get out of bed. She asked me to pick it up for him. I turned my back to her, bent over and mimed picking up an object. Mom seemed satisfied with my gesture, but what do I do now? Do I pretend Dad is there? Do I try to reorient her? How do you tell your mother that her husband of sixty-three years has been gone for a year and a half?

I decided to remind her gently that Dad wasn't with us. I choked back my tears as I told her. I observed a subtle shift in her awareness and then she softly said, "I know now, that you've told me."

As Death Nears

As the end gets closer, mottling of the extremities may occur. The heart is no longer pumping blood effectively and this poor circulation means blood pools in the nail beds, feet and hands giving them a bluish tinge, and they will feel cold to touch. Blood pressure often drops and changes occur in pulse—either slowing or increasing substantially. A slight fever is fairly common. The eyes of the patient may be semi-open or open but not seeing or focused on this world.

"Terminal agitation" may arise. This can be a difficult thing to see but often occurs as the final hours approach. Flailing and jerking may occur as well as the patient trying to get up to leave. Some medications can be used to provide calming, but generally, it has been suggested that this agitation is related to low oxygen in the blood, and not pain. The patient may be increasingly confused.

Breathing changes. The normal breathing may be replaced by a more intense gasping for air. The phrase "death rattle" refers to the secretions that can gather in the throat causing a rattling sound during respiration. This is not painful to the dying, but can feel uncomfortable for those at bedside. Often hospice nurses will provide *atropine* to lessen the congestion. As the end nears, breathing can become irregular with long pauses between inhalations. This apnea can be nerve-wracking for those keeping vigil; the patient may seem lifeless during a long pause and then take a gasp and continue to breathe.

Pastor Rob came to visit Mom today and give her communion and perform the Commendation for the Dying. We all communed with her, even 7-month-old Ellie. We sang, "Jesus Loves Me." We prayed. We shared. When we finished, she closed her eyes for a few moments, and we all thought, "Oh, God! She's gone!" Then she popped open her eyes, looked around at everyone and said, "Just kidding!" We didn't know whether to laugh or cry. Rob said, "Did she really just do that???" All along we thought she was in denial or didn't understand she was dying, but this proved she really did know what was happening, and she was comfortable enough with it to joke about it.

Emotionally and Spiritually

Several days or weeks before death several unusual behaviors may take place. The person may seem unresponsive as they detach from this world. It is common to see individuals picking at the bedclothes, sheets or just at the air, often stretching out as if to touch something or someone just out of reach.

Individuals may see deceased loved ones or "others" who are visible to no one else. These spirits come into the room and are solid and definite to the dying person. Your loved one may ask about these visitors or know intrinsically that they are there for a purpose. Whether you understand these apparitions as real or a hallucination is unimportant. **They are very real to the dying person.** There is no need to challenge these type of visions if they are not creating a danger for your loved one. Often it is a surprise who comes to the dying. One might expect to hear about a previously deceased spouse and learn that it is a great-aunt who is appearing!

If the patient becomes scared or hysterical due to hallucinations, end of life care can include certain anti-psychotic medications to help calm this. Mention this to the nurse or doctor.

───※───

2:15 am. "No Mom, you don't have to go to work today. You can stay in bed. Okay, I'll call her. She will understand. Don't worry, I will take care of it. It will be okay."

───※───

Preparing for Approaching Death

Sometimes, the body is ready to die, but there is "unfinished business" that seems to keep them on this plane. Whether or not a chaplain or loved one is able to resolve the conflict for your loved one, it can be helpful for the close family to "give permission" for them to die. Know that this is a final act of love for your parent, letting them know they will not be forgotten and that you will be okay. It may be as simple as saying "I love you," or "It's okay to go."

Death rarely follows a linear path, alerting you exactly to its timeline. Hospice nurses, social workers, and chaplains often remark with amazement that their patients were "in transition" or "active" for days or even two weeks. How can professionals not know? Each individual dies in his or her own time. Whether you believe it is a Higher Power that calls them home or unfinished business that keeps them on earth, it is a mystery that can't be answered. It can be confounding and exhausting for caregivers to begin to "vigil" only to have the parent rally.

For some, a visit from a loved one or being given "permission" to let go seems to allow them to release. However, just as likely is the scenario that they die only when their sweetheart leaves the room for a moment allowing them to go alone. Do they need that space to focus on the beyond or do they sense it is kinder for them to just slip away? In the bereavement field, we talk about being accompanied only to the edge of the bridge but having to cross it alone. Whether your loved one is by herself when their life here ends or whether she is surrounded by family, that bridge is theirs to cross.

April 17

As fragile crystal snowflakes gently blanket the earth, Kevin and I hold vigil, mindful that the end of mom's journey is drawing near. My brothers and our children and our dear friends gather and we wait and we watch; carefully measuring the time we have left. Minutes filled with chatting, reminiscing, singing, laughing, sighing. We hasten to satisfy the few requests she makes, and try to help her see through the cloud of confusion permeating her thoughts.

I am reminded of our childhood when the Watt family would come to visit on a holiday or summer vacation. Adults talking over coffee late into the night while cousins played and claimed a space to sleep on the basement floor. There were Grandma's cinnamon rolls and trips to the mountains. But mostly there was family; a celebration of our heritage. Each generation having its own personality, changing with the times. But tradition clings desperately to the present, fearful it will be forgotten with each passing year.

We are out of time. There will be no more calling her at 5:30 on Thanksgiving morning asking for turkey-roasting advice. There will be no more birthday cards with $5 tucked inside, no more lunch dates, no more concerts, no more pant-hemming. I will never again hear her voice sing hymns at church or watch her play with Colin and Ellie. And I will never see a Mickey Mouse or watch Downton Abbey without thinking of her.

My wise husband, who always sees the big picture, reassures me that in twenty years we will be able to look back on this—the time we walked with my mother at the end of her pilgrimage—and know we did the right thing. Even though we made mistakes, our intentions were good, and we did it for the right reasons.

I am deeply grateful for our beautiful hospice team, selfless friends and family who wait with us and come to help at a moment's notice, run errands, buy bird feeders, and help satisfy cravings. Pastors who are also friends, respite care, snow, forever friends, music that touches the heart, old T.V. shows, handyman-superheroes, brothers, nieces, nephews, grandbabies, cousins, bad jokes, symphony advice, CNA-manicurists who travel to your home. Brownie-making, flower-bringing, do-si-do-giving, book-making piano students, miniature snowmen, children's books, random conversation, guitar-serenades. My husband.

NOTES AND THOUGHTS

10

DEATH

This is an impossible time. We wait and watch and hold hands, but it doesn't ease the worry. I wish the world could just pause and wait with us while we hold our breath ... but time keeps going. —Cara

Are we ever really prepared for death? If you are caring for your loved one at home, you may want to know that at the time of death you will find no responsiveness, breathing or heartbeat, the eyes may be slightly open with the pupils fixed, and there may be a release of the bladder or bowels. The muscles relax and the jaw may open slightly; you will likely find your loved one's skin will droop and may look waxy. For most caregivers, there is a sense that the body remains but the essence of the person has gone.

You and your family members may wish to be with your loved one after death. For some, religious observances may dictate this. Your family might choose to sit with the deceased, dress the body or to light a candle in remembrance. There is no right way to handle this event. Older children may be encouraged but never forced to "say goodbye" to a relative. With children, they should be told the truth in simple terms and it should be explained that their loved one has died and is not just asleep. If your family has included younger kids in the time prior to death, saying goodbye after death can be a choice but never a requirement.

Children may be encouraged but never forced to "say goodbye."

If your loved one has been on hospice service you will have been instructed to first call hospice who will send a medical professional to confirm the death. Once the nurse comes to the home to assess for the absence of vital signs, she or he will contact the doctor of record to report the death and will call the coroner's office noting the hospice diagnosis for the cause of death. The nurse will also be responsible for destroying remaining narcotics that have been prescribed.

If you are not affiliated with a hospice and the death occurs at home you will likely call the coroner's office in your county. Calling the emergency services number, 911, will generally bring paramedics who will attempt resuscitation. If your loved one was at a facility at the time of death, they will help guide you through the process. If there is any question about the cause of death or possible neglect contributing to death, it is likely the coroner will be involved.

To arrange for the body to be removed, the family should follow:

- the coroner's instructions
- the information from the hospital or organ donation center
- the details provided by the mortuary or crematory you have selected
- the hospice team's directions

Death in a Hospital

The last time I saw Dad, he didn't open his eyes. He was lying in his hospital bed, breathing with the assistance of a bi-pap machine. He was suffering incurable pneumonia; his lungs extremely weak after living for years on oxygen with COPD. He had been sedated and restrained to prevent him from pulling at the lines and getting out of bed. I hated seeing his arms bound. I knew that he despised being told what to do. He viewed it as a violation of his freedom—and this was the extreme—he was being held against his will; a prisoner of his body, too ill to return to his home. He was only hours from death, and he had wanted to die in a familiar place, his wife by his side, among his treasures, where he was in control. The hospital could not release him. I could not help him. I failed. Indeed, I will carry that guilt with me until the end of my days.

I managed to rally my siblings and our spouses and children to his bedside. It was all I could do. We held

*Dad's hand. We talked gently to him. We comforted him. We joked. He always had such a hearty sense of humor and a boisterous laugh ... the joking in that moment was good. Mom had tried to lift his eyelids so Dad could see that we were all with him. "Oh, Grandma ... " Andrew said, adoringly. We chuckled, but now I realize the urgency of that playful, yet desperate act. We all wanted to see him, but she wanted to **see** him. She wanted him to see **her**.*

It is inspiring to see the family gather, play music, laugh and comfort each other. Even though this day has worn me thin, I will treasure these smiles and music for a long time.   —Cara

Theirs was a tumultuous marriage, to be sure; never hiding their annoyances from one another. Even so, she was sad. That, we saw in her eyes. Of course, she was sad. Sixty-three years they had been married. Sixty-three turbulent years. But they were companions, nonetheless. They withstood the storms. And there were storms. But there were calm moments, too. Moments of love, and happiness, and true joy. She didn't say much that night, nor did she release his hand. Her grip was immovable.

Dad summoned every bit of strength he could muster to say, "Goodbye." I had not known my father to be more loving and courageous than he was in that moment. It took everything he had left to give us those words. He loved his family more than anything. He was afraid to say it, but this, his final gift, transcended love.

Still holding his hand, Mom kissed him sweetly. She looked up at me, her eyes searching, bereft, forlorn … "I can't believe he's gone."

—⚬⚬⚬—

There are two likely scenarios if your loved one is in the hospital at the time of death—they are an admitted patient who dies or whose life support is disconnected or they arrive at the emergency department and are pronounced dead at that time. Hospitals have staff chaplains and social workers to help a family navigate this emotional and stressful event and offer resources. If a mortuary has not previously been chosen, the family will probably be informed that the patient's body may be kept in the morgue for up to several weeks if necessary while decisions are finalized.

When a patient is brought to the emergency department via ambulance, the EMTs will have likely tried to offer life-saving techniques such as CPR and defibrillation. This will continue at the hospital until such time as a medical doctor declares the patient dead. The attending nurse will contact the coroner's office as well as place a call to the local Organ Procurement Organization (OPO) to find out if there is a donor record on file. A chaplain will be called to offer comfort and provide or obtain information about organ donation. Note that even though your loved one may be advanced in age, certain types of organ donation are possible. It is important to alert the OPO within two hours of death so appropriate care can be taken. For more information on organ donation, go to www.organdonor.gov.

Why is the coroner called? In each state, the coroner's office has certain regulations around what might be considered a suspicious death. In most cases, the coroner's representative will simply ask the family about the circumstances around the end of life and will examine the body at the hospital. In certain cases, the coroner will remove the body to the coroner's office to examine it there. The body will most likely be able to be released to the mortuary within a few days and the family is responsible for telling the coroner which mortuary will handle the funeral or cremation. The mortuary or funeral home will be responsible for transporting the body from the coroner's office to their location.

Should your loved one be on life support and the doctor feels there is no hope of recovery, the chaplain, social worker, and nurse will probably be present when the doctor has this discussion with the family. Prior to removing life support, a chaplain can aid in performing rituals or can call for other clergy to do so. The decision around a mortuary should be decided before death.

It is worth noting that the MDPOA's role will legally cease at time of death. It is the next of kin who can make decisions after that time. For many, these two roles are played by one person, but should your loved one be in a medical facility at the time of death and decisions are not finalized, the order of next of kin may be the "personal representative," spouse, adult children or adult siblings.

Finally, if the death takes place in a hospital, you may be invited to attend a memorial service for family members whose loved ones have died over the past months. These services can be moving and healing and are another opportunity to transition from mourner to bereaved. Hospices also provide their own memorial services where families and staff can remember and honor those who have died.

Should you require financial assistance for burial, contact your local County Department of Social Services for information. Additionally, if the deceased was in the military or was the spouse of an eligible military veteran, there may be benefits available for burial including internment at a VA national cemetery. Contact the Department of Veterans Affairs for full information.

—◦◦◦◦—

This is the first time I've been alone in the house since mom moved in—it feels surreal.

Everyone returned to their lives, and their obligations, and their routines, and I returned to ... what? For the last fourteen months, my life consisted of serving, guessing, crying, defending, succumbing. I didn't remember who I was or what my purpose was supposed to be. I felt more deeply alone than I thought ever possible. How do you navigate living without a mommy?

So now, I am faced with quite the dichotomy. Do I choose the desire to process in solitude, or the companionship that allows me to avoid contemplating my heartache?

—◦◦◦◦—

Immediately Afterwards ...

Once calls have been made to family, religious leader and friends to alert them to the death and plans are in place for the disposition of the body, the first few days are usually consumed with arrangements and mourning. Most funeral homes will provide the family with a list of organizations that should be contacted following the death, funeral or memorial service.

Death certificates are usually obtained through the funeral home. It is advisable to estimate how many you will need based on the institutions that will require legal proof of death. If you later need more, you can contact the Vital Statistics Department in the county where death occurred of the Department of Public Health, Vital Records Office.

There are very few things that must be attended to in the first days following a death. Most paperwork cannot be started until copies of the death certificate are provided. The settling of the estate may take weeks, months, or even years, so it is advisable to be as methodical as you can.

You will not need to dispose of clothes or possessions immediately. (However, if your loved one was in a care facility you should make certain of how long the facility will give you to clean out a room/apartment before charging for additional days.) If at all possible, take some time to decide whether this is the right time to dispose of items. Favorite clothes may hold special memories, jacket pockets may have reminders, and a worn garment may keep alive the scent of person. It can be an emotionally charged exercise to go through a closet, and you may not be ready to donate or discard items. If you have the ability to wait for a calmer time to go through personal items, do so.

———

The memorial service is over. Everyone has gone home, but my home is filled with her. They all get to move on, but I still have to tie up all the loose ends. Her dirty laundry is still sitting in her hamper. Her medication is still in the kitchen cabinet. Her glasses and hearing aid on her nightstand. Her Mickey Mouse laying alone, on the foot of her bed ...

They all get to move on, but I still have to tie up all the loose ends.

Everything that remains of my parents' lives is stacked in a few boxes in the corner of mom's bedroom. How do one's possessions constitute a life? Their lingering love, their passion, their memory, sorted and stored. Only as long as someone cares enough to remember them, will their existence be true. How long until they are not thought of every day, how long before they are not remembered, before no one knows their name?

NOTES AND THOUGHTS

11

GRIEF

You can't bypass grief—
you have to walk through it.

Y ou can't bypass grief—you have to walk through it. The pain of grief lessens over time, but it never fully goes away. This is a blessing and a curse. We surely do not want to forget, but the pain is hard to bear. Generally, grief lingers longer than our society acknowledges. The idea that a worker in the United States gets three days for bereavement would be laughable if it weren't so sad.

Grief is not a straight line but may instead mimic a pendulum swinging from side to side, leaving the bereaved vacillating from feeling hopeful about the future to being "stuck" in mourning. Try to be patient with yourself during this time of unique experience. Grief looks and feels different for every individual. Your family members, and you within your family will each have a slightly different experience and will react to it in varying ways.

Dr. Alan Wolfelt, a nationally-known grief counselor, author, and educator notes that mourning is paradoxical: When we try to ignore the pain, we don't heal. Thus, you have to fully acknowledge what you have lost and the significance of death and change; you will need to recognize and embrace the grief and darkness discovering what it has to teach you; and, you must learn to recount memories, ritual, disappointments in order to name your gratitude and begin to move forward. Loss is complex and rushing through the process may extend the healing time.

As you and your loved one prepare for the rituals that make up mourning, know that going through the motions may be the most you can hope for. You may feel a sense of unreality or numbness. While some folks find comfort in taking charge of the details surrounding a funeral or burial, others may just withdraw. Where ever you are on your journey, expect it to change and last longer than you expect.

Grief is unpredictable. It is intense. It's mean. It's intimate. Grief pesters. Grief doesn't care that you are in a rush or in a public place ... like when you're walking into ACE Hardware and you see a kindly, balding hippie escorting his thin, Levis-rocking, elderly mother into the store. She stops to look at the flowers and he waits patiently as she admires them. Grief mocks you in this everyday moment, subtly pointing out that this guy still has his mother and he's doing it right.

Or when you are in your mother's room trying to find a place for her wedding dress to live and you see the last few touchable pieces of her life sitting in a corner. Grief takes you by the hand and says, "We're not finished." You can still smell her perfume ...

Or when you are doing the laundry and one of her Mickey Mouse socks falls from a towel. Grief toys with you.

Or when you are cooking dinner and you can hear her slight Nebraskan twang saying, "Just a little bit ... "

Grief taps you on the shoulder and reminds you of who you are, where you came from, and who you struggle to be.

Grief drapes you in cottony gauze; protecting your wound, yet allowing you still to breathe. Grief is mean, but it is a means.

During the first few days and weeks after a death, you may find yourself with physical and emotional complaints that are scary and unexpected: no one tells you how strongly the body reacts to grief:

- Uncontrolled crying or bursts of grief that come on without warning
- Generalized weakness or extreme fatigue
- Sleep disturbance—sleeping too much or insomnia
- Food issues—gorging or inability to eat at all
- Pain or feeling pressure in the chest (if this does not subside quickly this should be checked by a doctor)
- Shortness of breath
- A knot in the stomach or tightness in the throat
- Dizziness, headaches or noise sensitivity

- Additionally, your emotional and cognitive abilities are jumbled. You may experience:
- Inability to concentrate or remember things for weeks
- Lack of motivation
- Difficulty making decisions or organizing
- Confusion or a sense of disconnect from reality
- Tension and anxiety
- Feelings of abandonment, sadness or depression

How do you cope? Start by acknowledging that these emotions are real and overwhelming. Death loss—even when expected—can feel like a huge piece of you is missing. Rely on what brings you comfort: snuggling in a familiar blanket, taking a walk in the park, watching a favorite movie, sipping a calming tea, relaxing in a bubble bath, taking a nap. In order to take care of yourself through this time, it is important to try to eat nutritiously (small, more frequent meals may be helpful), attempt regular sleep habits, and do moderate exercise as you're able. Don't expect too much from yourself. It may be days or weeks before you feel productive. It is also not unusual for the caregiver to get sick after the death; after all the strain and sleeplessness around dying and mourning, the body is worn out.

—————∞—————

When your body needs nourishment, but you're not hungry—nothing is appetizing, nothing is right. You can't sleep, you can't wake up. You can't cry, you can't smile. You want to talk but you can't formulate the words. Or thought.

Your house is falling apart. You know you need help but you can't ask. Your spirit has vanished. You are empty.

Isn't there someone who can take over for you? Someone who can step inside your skin and let you fade into the darkness for a while. Someone to do your dishes, sweep your floor, bake some cookies, and do your dead mother's laundry.

People keep checking in, but do they really want to help? They say, "If you need anything, just ask." But the asking is too hard. It is a cruel request to force an empty spirit to ask for help.

We tussle with a lingering sense of urgency even though there is nothing pressing. This crisis has become our story. We survived, but more, we are still surviving.

There is no timeline you need to follow either for change or for grief. Everyone grieves differently.

Grief is Unique

The expression of grief varies by culture, geography, family, and gender as well as the unique history and personality of the bereaved. Men and women both need to remind themselves that crying is an appropriate and healthy expression of grief. The physical action of crying helps to expel built up tension in your body, releases stress hormones, and provides an emotional release for the loss you're feeling. However, if you aren't weepy that can be your "normal." Allow yourself the full range of emotions.

Whenever possible, put off major life decisions such as moving to a different residence, changing jobs, etc. for the first year after your loss. Well-meaning friends or relatives may try to encourage you to "get away from the memories." Don't allow others to take over or rush you through these decisions – you can make these decisions little by little as you're ready.

Triggers are everywhere. From the knick knacks on the shelf or the smell of a certain aftershave or a specific time of day, memories can flood your senses at any moment. Even when you feel you are more or less in control and you are calmly going about your day, the reminders come unbidden.

Grief and Children

There are many good books to help explain death and loss to children. Although the continuum of explanation will be based on their age, comprehension, and their relationship with the deceased, the death should be discussed and normalized. Kids respond to death in as many ways as adults, but there are some generalizations that may help as they try to make sense of what they see and feel. The child's school counselor and teacher should be notified of the death. If school grades drop, behaviors change, or sleep is disturbed, consider consulting a play therapist or grief counselor who works with teens.

1. Children want to know about their own safety and security. When a loved one dies,

they wonder who might die next and who will take care of them. Answer them honestly, but assure them that there are a number of people who are able to care for them.

2. The expression of grief is healthy for them to see. Acknowledge the loss and the emotion that it engenders. "Mommy is sad and is crying because she misses Nana."

3. Use simple language that they can understand and avoid phrases like "gone to sleep" or "gone away." Children can take these phrases literally and become afraid of going to sleep or worry that loved ones are being hidden from them. Saying a person died establishes a permanence. If your family professes a belief in an afterlife, explain heaven; don't expect a child to have an understanding of this.

4. Younger children's attention span for death and sadness can be quite short. Often they will be sad one minute and then wish to play. This is normal and doesn't reflect their feelings of love.

5. Up to about the age of 10, children engage in "magical thinking." They may blame themselves for the death or feel their loved one got sick because of something they did. Explain living and dying as a natural process.

6. Teens may not wish to engage with the family around death. Allow teenagers to have time

with their peers and be open to grief groups and weekend camps such as Camp Erin (nationally sponsored by the Moyer Foundation) which provides a safe space to share emotions. As they are willing, encourage journaling, art, sports, and favorite activities. Offer opportunities for them to participate in grief rituals so they know they are included.

7. Offer photographs and mementos to remember your loved one and talk about favorite memories.

Tim called today. Today is Tuesday. Tuesday is the day Tim calls to chat with Mom. I sometimes forget that they lost their mom, too.

Many bereaved individuals begin to feel guilty about how much their grief is intruding on their life. Grieving takes longer than anyone can imagine. However, if after several weeks or months, you are not noticing any improvement in your ability to cope or finding a balance between mourning the past and looking to the future, then you may want to consult with a grief counselor.

Beyond the expected emotions, others may creep in that surprise us. Guilt, real or imagined, is a normal part of grief and may present itself in thoughts like, "if only ... " Try to express these feelings and learn to forgive yourself. Anger is another emotion that can catch us off guard and may then initiate feelings of guilt. Journaling, support groups, therapy and processing your emotions with close friends and loved ones may be how you get through this.

If writing is your preferred style, you might consider penning a letter to your loved one sharing your emotions. The act of putting the words on paper/computer can be cathartic. Some find comfort in sending "observations of gratitude" to the universe by way of safely burning or compiling a group of notes stored in a special vessel.

⸺⸺

I am experiencing what is referred to as, "Complicated Grief"—A state in which the survivor "remains stuck in an unresolved and long-lasting response to a significant loss." This doesn't seem to be caused by inadequate coping after Mom's death, but rather by the hopelessness of the relationship we shared. Her illness, our respective stubbornness, and her ultimate death robbed us of any chance we had to treasure the time we had left and share in the intimacy of death. As a result, I have a one-way mental dialogue looping over and over in my head: "Why are you staring at me? What can I get you? What do you want? Please, just tell me what you want!"

In the days before her death, at the suggestion of mom's nurse, I jotted things down in a notebook that I wanted to remember: things mom said, things others said, tasks I needed to complete, questions I needed to ask the hospice staff, things that upset or worried me, people I wanted to thank, mom's quickly changing physical status. ...

When her symptoms began escalating rapidly, and her needs became more intense, I began to feel increasingly fretful and isolated. So tired. So much chaos. I just wanted to sleep and be alone. For every moment I craved companionship during our journey, I craved aloneness now, even more.

When you are grieving, people think you should not be alone. They think they need to keep you company or to make you smile, or hug you, or give you their shoulder to cry on. But all that attention, at least for me, kept me from actually experiencing my grief and moving toward my healing. I didn't want hugs. I didn't want to confide in anyone or cry on their shoulder. I wanted to be alone. I wanted rest. I experienced extreme and profound exhaustion. The internet told me this was the "lethargy of grief," and it was normal. Sounded reasonable to me. So after they'd gone, I turned off my phone, locked the door, and slept.

NOTES AND THOUGHTS

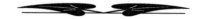

12

OBITUARIES, EULOGIES, AND MEMORIALS

Thank you, everyone, for your love and support. We are overwhelmed by the numerous posts, emails, and texts we have received from our friends and family. They have been a great source of comfort during our time of grief. We are truly blessed.

W hat can be said about funerals? In the recent past in the United States, many families have chosen to forgo this ceremony, opting for a memorial service at a later date or a celebration of life. While certain cultures and religions have strict guidelines for end of life practices, many Americans find themselves at loose ends trying to figure out when to scatter the ashes or gather friends and family.

As a rule, having some sort of service or remembrance within the first weeks can provide a sense of forward motion. Once a death occurs, mourners may wish to cocoon themselves in a state of disbelief, not feeling strong enough to move forward. On the other hand, if the service is delayed for months, wounds that have begun healing organically may be broken wide open again. Planning and participating in a formal goodbye is a healthy way to acknowledge the loss and take the next steps into the future.

Laughter at the funeral can break the solemnity and can also release tears that are trapped.

As a grief counselor, I often focus on helping families create special memorials. Are there songs or mementos that must be included? Is there a particular charity that your loved one would wish to support? Is there a location that is important? If this is a small family gathering, what do you want this service to provide to you?

Writing an obituary or a eulogy is one way to remain connected to your loved one. While many funeral homes will help with the obituary, and a life story may be composed by a clergyperson after interviewing family, it can be therapeutic to gather this information prior to the death. Most eulogies are delivered by family members and usually include funny memories or stories that offer a glimpse into the life of the deceased. Laughter at the funeral can break the solemnity and can also release tears that are trapped, but if that is not your family's style, then keep it simple and honest.

While obituaries are often written immediately after death, it can be helpful to write the life story as your loved one wishes to see it, prior to their dying. This can be a task assigned to someone other than the caregiver. For a host of reasons, some psychological and some superstitious, it is probably most helpful NOT to include a date, location, or service information on any draft document! For families whose loved one led a rich and varied life of service which will be detailed in the obituary, it is a good idea to fact-check dates, locations, and titles before coming under a publishing deadline. As it has become the norm to charge for newspaper obituaries, the family might want to discuss the length and content. Will there be a photo? If so, who will select this? How many great-grandchildren will be listed by name?

Writing an Obituary

Simple guidelines for writing an obituary or a biography sketch:

- Full name of the deceased including parents' names, maiden name or nickname
- Funeral service information
- Date and location of birth, marriage, death
- Schools attended
- Military service including rank and branch of service
- Major employment or business name
- Membership in organizations
- Special interests, honors and awards
- Surviving relations
- Charities or websites where donations may be made "in lieu of flowers"

Because most print newspapers will charge for an obituary, make clear how much detail should be shared in print or if the obituary may be shared online, through a mortuary's website, or simply in a program that is distributed at a memorial or funeral service.

Cremains, Graveyards, Memorials

Your family and your loved one may have very specific wishes about burial. For those who follow a religious tradition, burial, cremation or funerals can have strict dictates which provide structure. When there are no guidelines, it is worth noting that different family members may want to have a say in the disposition of the remains.

Cremains—the cremated remains of the body—can be returned to the family in an urn, box or memorialized in jewelry or decorative items. If your family is going to scatter or divide cremains among survivors, make these plans specific. Placing cremains in a garden or a permanent resting place will be much different than bringing home your loved one in an urn. Some family members select a beautiful urn and display it within a shrine at home with photos and special mementos. Other families keep the cremains tucked away until they choose to scatter them. This is strictly a personal choice.

If your loved one wanted to be buried in a cemetery, you will discover there are some regulations about burials that vary from state and location and within religious cemeteries. Is a vault required? Is there perpetual care? Can cremains be buried? Can multiple family members' cremains be comingled?

If a funeral has been prepaid, there may still be costs associated with moving or storing the body or engraving the tombstone, for example. Check with the funeral director to learn what is covered.

—⊷⊶—

Good News! We Found Dad!

When it was time to pick out an urn for Dad's cremains at the meeting with the cremation service, Kevin jokingly suggested we put them in one of the Avon Aftershave Cars that Mom collected for him. Mom loved the idea, so I retrieved them from storage where they were packed in an Orville Redenbacher Popcorn box, washed them out, and took them to the crematory. The instructions were that he was to be divided into the cars so Mom and my brothers and I could each have one.

When Mom and I returned to the crematorium to pick Dad up, we discovered they only placed a dusting of his ashes in each of the cars and the bulk of the ashes rested in a free plastic urn that they provided (which really wasn't an urn, but a plastic box, enclosed in a cardboard box, slid into a cardboard sleeve). The "urn" and the cars were returned to us in the Orville Redenbacher Popcorn box. When Mom saw it she laughed and said, "What's he doing in that box??!!" I guess she had forgotten we decided to use the cars and thought it would be just like him to choose to rest for eternity in a popcorn box.

I remember watching Dad shave in the mornings when I was little; buzzing his face with his electric razor. Sometimes he would tickle my cheek lightly with the buzzing razor. I liked that. After he shaved, he would pour aftershave from one of those Avon cars into his hands, rub them together, and slap his face. I didn't know why he had to slap himself. He could have just dabbed his wrists. That's what Mom did when she wanted to smell good, and I'm sure her method was much less painful.

Mom purchased the cars from the Avon Lady and after a few years, he owned the entire collection. He even built a special display shelf for them. They were cool, and I had some favorites, but they held some of the most pungent scents you ever smelled. Dad sold most of the cars at a garage sale when they moved out of our childhood home on Dudley Street, but he kept a few and rationed his stinky cologne usage for when he and Mom went out.

After Dad's funeral, some of the cars and the popcorn box came to my house, where it sat temporarily in our bedroom. The urn went with mom to their apartment where it sat, perched on the dresser.

In times of chaos, your brain does amazing things to protect you from stress.

When we moved Mom into our house from the apartment, Dad supervised the moving process from his place on the dresser in the plastic urn; making sure everything was packed just so. He did, after all, like to be in control. (I think it was really that no one wanted to pack him away in a U-Haul box with the Mickey Mouse collection or the con-

*tents of the underwear drawer.) Anyway, we wouldn't have
wanted him to get lost in the move, or worse, spilled.*

*When it was time to carry the dresser out, he was
placed on the table. When the table had to go, he was given
a cozy spot on the floor. He was moved from spot to spot
until everything had been loaded onto the truck. When we
made our final pass-through, scanning the apartment for
any remaining items, there was Dad, sitting on the floor. I
was already juggling his portable oxygen tank, a rug from
the bathroom, and the gold trash can that always sat on the
floor by his nightstand, but I picked him up and wrapped
him carefully in a plastic bag, and placed him gently into
the trash can. "It will only be for the ride home," I said to
myself, thinking of the inappropriateness of putting him in
a trash can, but I'd hold him on my lap once I got into the
car.*

*In times of chaos, your brain does amazing things
to protect you from stress. In my mind, the ashes in the
cars and the ashes in the urn were all resting together in
the Orville Redenbacher Popcorn box in our bedroom. All
was in the same place. I discovered however, that sharing
our marital bedroom with my father's ashes was creepy and
totally disrupted our bedroom's Feng Shui. So, I made plans
to give him a place of honor in Mom's room. When I picked
the box up however, it felt surprisingly light and I realized
the plastic urn wasn't with the Avon cars. I had lost Dad.
Shit. I lost my Dad. How do you lose your father's ashes???
Mortified, I called my brothers to tell them I lost our father.
I had promised to take care of him, and I lost him.*

*Kevin and I began searching. We were almost
certain he was lost in the move. When you have nearly a
dozen folks volunteering to move your parent's things into*

nearly half a dozen locations, it is impossible to keep track of every item. In the midst of the confusion, the urn had disappeared. Kevin was determined though, and did not give up the search. Dad would reveal his location eventually. Finally, his whereabouts were discovered. It was a matter of "Last out, first in," (LOFI) in which Dad was the last out of the apartment and first into (gulp) storage, having been mistaken for a can full of miscellaneous items.

Where did we find him? The shed ... My father's ashes had been stored in a plastic urn, enclosed in a cardboard box, slid into a cardboard sleeve, wrapped in a plastic bag, placed into a golden trash can, and unknowingly tucked into the back of our shed for longer than I want to admit. The good news is that Dad was found, and he and Mom are quietly dreaming, side by side, in her room for the time being.

NOTES AND THOUGHTS

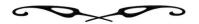

13

BEREAVEMENT DOESN'T REALLY END

You discover she held onto your father's yellow windbreaker, and you find two butterscotch candies and a starlight mint in his left pocket. You know he tucked them away to give to his grandchildren.

For many people who are grieving, there is the uncomfortable discovery that the actual death is much more than missing the individual who died. You suddenly have no role to play as a caregiver and you may no longer feel useful. While you were once part of a couple and maybe part of a social group, you now feel like a third wheel. In some cases, the loss of the family home or splitting up of heirlooms among siblings leaves a hollow feeling.

In their book, *All Our Losses, All Our Griefs*, Mitchell and Anderson write about the different types of losses:

- Material—loss of physical objects
- Relationship—close relationships of all types which are gone
- Intra-psychic—loss of an emotionally important image of oneself or what might have been
- Functional—loss of body part, muscular or neurological control
- Role—loss of a significant social role
- Systemic—disconnect with a system that supported you

When grief counselors talk about a new normal, this is what they are referring to: the bereaved person will need to discover their new identity and a new relationship with the outside world—an internal lens has shifted. Imagine having surgery on your leg and having to relearn to walk. You will feel pain, discover limitations, force yourself to do exercises to strengthen your muscles, and even after you are healed, you may walk with a limp or notice a scar. Every once in a while you will recall and acknowledge life before your surgery or your previous abilities. This is grief.

⸺⸜⸝⸻

My new motto is: "One thing a day." Sometimes the only thing you can accomplish in one day is removing a few items of clothing from your mother's closet. It might take you two days to fold and bag them, or it might take a whole week.

You will chuckle at the fact that there is an entire bag devoted to sweater vests ... After placing the bags in the car for donation, you might turn around and pull them right back out again. A week later, after rescuing a sweater vest you think might make a nice pillow cover, and a skirt you imagine will make a lovely scarf, you ask your husband to carry the bags back out to the car for you. You drive them to the donation place, take a deep breath, and hand them to the person accepting donations. One thing a day. It's (not) so hard ...

───────

Holidays

The first year is often the worst. Which is not to say that other years are easy! Still, getting through the first birthday, anniversary, Mother's Day, Father's Day, Memorial Day, death anniversary ... these dates can fill you with dread. Your body may take over anticipatory grief for you. Often, before you realize why you are feeling so low, your body has responded to the month around the death. I encourage you to plan for these emotion-laden days. What will you do to honor the memory of your parent? Will you toast her memory at dinner? Take a drive to look over a favorite vista? Is a visit to the gravesite appropriate? Light a memorial candle? Take yourself on a vacation?

Holidays generally conjure up memories of feasting and fun, celebrations and ceremony, laughter and loving. But what happens after a loved one has died and you are not sure how you will get through the upcoming holidays? For many people, the anticipation of any holiday brings anxiety and a sense of dread for the changes that are sure to be obvious at this time.

───────

My parents gave us extra challenges over the holidays. I always dreaded them. Yet here I am facing my first Thanksgiving without Mom or Dad, and I am sad.

Dad has been gone a little over two years. I found myself not dwelling on his absence much while I was caring for mom. I never really had a chance to process his death with all the responsibility that came with her care. A distraction that in retrospect was probably a blessing ... Mom was my connection to him, and now that she is gone too, I'm feeling a bit pensive and hollow.

It would not be Thanksgiving if our basement didn't flood. This was usually caused by Mom putting potato peels down our disposal. We learned to make sure all vegetables were stripped of their skin before she entered the house. We also learned to pick walnuts out of our Thanksgiving meal. Mom was of the belief that a Thanksgiving dish was incomplete without walnuts. She threw them in the sweet potatoes, the stuffing, the cranberries, the salad, in the pies, garnished the relish tray with them, and finally, piled the nut bowl high with unshelled walnuts and gave them a place of honor on the coffee table for everyone to snack on while they waited for dinner to be served. I am not a walnut fan, so one by one, I replaced her recipes with my own, sans walnuts.

Dad had lots of rules. Mostly unspoken, until you broke one, then you were made fully aware of your transgression. Sometimes, however, you didn't find out that you'd broken a rule until you showed up on his "anything anyone has ever done to wrong me" list. If you did end up on this list, you were there for life. He never forgave, and he never forgot.

His rules included, but were not limited to:

1. *He and Mom must receive their invitation at least three months prior to the event.*
2. *They will show up early.*
3. *They will leave early. (Because Dad's oxygen was running low from showing up early.)*
4. *If Mom and Dad come to your house for a gathering, you are still expected to go to their house later for the "real celebration."*
5. *Everyone must wear their holiday best. Dad usually wore his red sweater.*
6. *Get a haircut. (If you are male.) (Females should always have long hair.)*
7. *Don't talk too much, but don't be shy. Don't look at him without smiling, and above all else, Do. Not. Disagree. With. Dad.*
8. *Eggnog is best served diluted with milk over ice, then spiked with Rum. Lots of Rum.*
9. *The holidays are coming, it's time for Dad to clean out his cupboards and make "junk" from all his leftover cereals, crackers, bags of chips, and cans of nuts.*

"One thing a day"

For the first time in my life, I don't have to worry about myself or my family doing (or not doing) something that would land us on Dad's list. I don't have to worry about the basement flooding, or picking walnuts out of my food. Nor will I get to hear Dad greet everyone with the nicknames he's given them all. I won't see his face light up as his grandsons shake his hand and say, "Hi Grandpa!" I won't see him give his grandchildren hugs then sneak them a butterscotch or a Starlight Mint from his pocket before dinner. I won't hear the "whoosh-cha, whoosh-cha" of his portable oxygen helping him to breathe, or smile at his hearty laugh. I won't have to worry about him telling an inappropriate joke, or if the cat will trigger a bronchial spasm. I won't have to find a job for Mom to do that doesn't involve peeling vegetables ...

There will be two empty places at our table this year. I am regretful. I am mournful. I am relieved. How can relief be so brutal?

Set Realistic Goals

Spend some time thinking about what you can handle. Have a conversation with family members or friends so that concerns can be addressed and communicate clearly what your wishes for the holidays are. There may be some members who need to observe certain traditions which you may not feel up to. Know that it isn't going to be easy, but you don't need to participate in every aspect. You can say "no." Simplify. Make a list of things you think you can manage, don't want to do, and what you'd like to change.

For example, will it be too painful to decorate the inside of the house? Is decorating the outside of the house something you'd enjoy? Perhaps you'd like to skip baking for the neighborhood. If shopping for gifts or even exchanging gifts is too burdensome, make other plans. For some, writing a holiday letter is too difficult.

Others may find great comfort or great discomfort attending religious services. If visiting family and friends is overwhelming, give yourself permission to skip this.

Recognize that the holidays can be exhausting. For those who are grieving a loss, the emotional and physical toll can be overwhelming. Stay well rested, drink water, keep expenses to a minimum, accept your limitations, accept help, and know that changes in routine can be a blessing in disguise. You will be able to handle more and things may be easier next year.

Include Your Grief

While your loved one may not be physically present, we can keep the memories present and real. Ignoring the absence will create a tension that will add stress. Consider some of the following:

- Make a memorial display – perhaps decorate a framed photo with holiday décor or a pillow made of a favorite flannel shirt
- Make or purchase small gifts in memory of the person who died
- Create a special ritual that acknowledges the loss, like lighting a candle that burns throughout the day.
- Reach out for companionship; alone time is fine, isolation is not healthy
- Start a new holiday tradition, perhaps going out of town
- Offer a toast, a song, or a prayer in memory of your loved one
- Allow yourself to mourn the loss for a peri-

od of time each day, then resolve to do one
thing that puts you in a holiday mood

It can be helpful to remind yourself that even
through the worst of the grief, your loved one probably
didn't wish you to be in pain. They likely wanted to be
remembered with joy.

April 20

*Today is one year since Mom passed from here to
there. That day seems so distant, yet so present. Our cousins,
friends, brothers, sister-in-law, nieces and nephew, and our
children all gathered to say goodbye. It was a day of light and
life, and love. We had pizza delivered. I remember thinking
that pizza restaurant probably thought we were having a
4-20 party, but when I saw that Patrick, Jayme's friend who
works there, had penned a note of encouragement on the
box, I knew the light surrounding us was brilliant and pure.*

*Mom was richly and warmly blanketed in love, and
Kevin and I abundantly supported by our friends and family.
We will never be able to adequately express our gratitude to
those who have supported us throughout our journey.*

*I took some time yesterday to read through the
condolences we had received during that time and became
utterly overwhelmed by the outpouring of love and com-
passion we received. Then I threw all but three of the cards
away. I feel a need to be connected to that time, but also an
urge to begin to disconnect from it. Moving forward takes
action.*

*Of the three I kept, one was from mom's best friend
Betty, with whom I feel a connection to mom's life before*

us, one from Kevin's student who honored his request for "un-sympathy" as sympathy strangely made it unbearable to cope at times, and the card I received from Molly's kids who had hoped that mom could take care of me in heaven and that somehow they could make it up to me. Children are so perfectly sweet and innocent. The three link the past, the present and the future; hope, humor, and protection. In my heart I have tucked away every word from the cards I threw away and the few I have kept, and will use them as a balm for my heart when it aches.

Alison very wisely advised me in a comment to one of my posts last year that I would grow from this experience, and indeed I have. Of all I have learned about myself, my family, my community, and my mother, I believe the most important is honesty. Honesty simplifies life. I feel so strongly about this that I will say it again, honesty simplifies life.

People cannot read your mind. If you want something, you need to ask for it. Just ask. Need a bird feeder? Bananas? Toilet paper? Ask. Need company, a prayer, an apology, or a hug? Don't assume, ask. How about a joke to lighten your day? You WILL receive jokes. Lots and lots of really bad jokes. Almost always your help is a just breath away. Hot sauce fairies and essential oil angels are real, my friends. All you need to do is ask.

I also learned that grief is not a bad thing. Grief is not mental illness or weakness of character. Grief does not have an expiration date. And no one, no one, has the right to monitor the duration or intensity of your grief. What is grief then? Grief is love. Plain and simple. Grief is connection. Grief is your link to that which you cannot physically touch or hold. Grief allows you to cling with heart and mind *for as long as your memory will allow. Grief is love. Warm, sweet, downy love.*

I am taking an uncharacteristic day off for myself today. Kind of a reward for making it through the months and months of care-giving, followed by a year of recovery from care-giving. I haven't watched it since she died, but to feel closer to mom today, I have the television playing her favorite, Downton Abbey. Pot roast and potatoes are on the stove for dinner as a reminder of Mom's usual request for "meat" when I made my grocery list. I have taken this time to empty my mind (hold your jokes, please) and allow myself to focus on Mom, and Dad, and our journey to this moment.

NOTES AND THOUGHTS

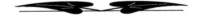

14

SUPPORTING THE MOURNER

It's not hard to talk about death these days. But when she said, "I'm so sorry about your mother. I've seen a lot of loss," my eyes well up with tears. Spritely 106-year-old Grandma Cora, alone in her generation—"But I have you," she says. Her words bring me comfort.

If you are the support person for someone who is grieving, you have an important role. For the bereaved, emotions may be all over the map and they may not know what they need. You may be afraid of intruding or making the person feel even worse. Even when you can't find the right words, a hug or comforting nod may be yours to give. Grief has no timeline and each individual will grieve in a unique way so expect grieving to last longer than anyone expects. Here are some guidelines to help you navigate this time.

The mourner may need to relive the circumstances around the death and process the experience again and again. You can listen and be empathic. They may feel lethargic and unable to participate in routine activities. You can be understanding. They may weep at inopportune moments. You can provide the tissues and no judgment. Acknowledge their unique pain without trying to wipe it away or compare it to anyone else's loss.

———⟨∞⟩———

Things I have learned from caregiving and grieving:

1. *It will be nothing like you imagined.*
2. *You will learn things about yourself you never knew before.*
3. *You will learn things about the person you cared for you never knew before.*
4. *You will use more bad words than you've ever used in your life.*
5. *Your spouse is your rock.*
6. *You will stay up way, way, way too late so you can have time alone.*
7. *Your friends and family and even complete strangers want to help you. Let them.*
8. *People's kindness will humble you and make you cry.*
9. *Be honest. Be patient. Be genuine. Hold fast. But also, give in.*
10. *Have a sense of humor.*
11. *Your best is good enough.*
12. *Say, "Thank you, and I Love You." Every. Single. Day.*

13. *Pace yourself. It's a marathon.*

14. *Your spouse is your rock.*

15. *Lysol wipes and latex gloves will be your best friends.*

16. *Jobs that normally take you 15 minutes to complete will literally take you all day. Not even kidding.*

17. *Ding Dongs are the perfect comfort food.*

18. *You will gain weight.*

19. *Sometimes you just have to turn off the baby monitor.*

20. *When you say, "Watt," your dishes get done.*

21. *Everyone grieves in their own way in their own time.*

22. *The first nap after a year of running on adrenaline is perfect.*

23. *Turn off your phone when you need to sleep.*

24. *There is never a wrong time for family and friends to pop in and "hold your cup."*

25. *People will say the wrong thing thinking they are being helpful. Forgive them, love them, and ignore the stupid things they say. Don't punch them in the throat.*

26. *Indeed, you are in the presence of the Lord when a member of the hospice team enters your home. Grace personified.*

27. *Your spouse is your rock.*

28. *Keep a "Hospital Kit" handy for when you have to sit for hours in the emergency room with your*

> parent. (phone charger, hoodie, Ding Dongs, Diet Coke, change of clothes for parent and medication list.)
>
> 29. When you think you can't do it anymore, you find out you're wrong. You have more strength than you know, and you see it through to the end.
>
> 30. Read the guest book. You won't remember who attended the funeral.
>
> 31. Be nice to your FedEx, UPS and USPS delivery people; you will be shopping online a lot.
>
> 32. Don't expect everyone to be sympathetic.
>
> 33. Trust your instincts.

When at all possible, avoid trite expressions that mean well, but can be hurtful for the newly bereaved. Noting you are "so sorry" may be all one can do. Do not try to find the magic words to eliminate the pain—there are none. If the bereaved acknowledges that their loved one is "not suffering anymore," validating that is very appropriate. However, telling someone their loved one "is in a better place," when that individual is not a believer in an afterlife and is just missing his or her parent greatly, may just exacerbate feelings of loss, guilt, and isolation.

These are a few suggestions of activities that say "I don't know exactly how to help, but I care and I am here for you."

- Call from time to time to check in
- Use the deceased's name and share memories

- Help make a list of chores that you can help with
- Drop off food (or bring food home)—don't wait to be asked
- Invite them out for a walk, a cup of coffee, breakfast, or a movie
- Send a card, make a donation or write a letter sharing memories
- Recognize that a refusal may simply indicate that the bereaved is not yet ready to engage

Particularly when the death is not expected or comes sooner than expected, the emotions can be extreme. Denial, guilt, anger, frustration, blame, acceptance, regret, and hopelessness can come at any time. Let your loved one know you are there for support. The bereaved often blame themselves for some omission in care. A grief counselor can help with this if it becomes a prolonged obsession, but a friend might remember the phrase, "You did what you could at the time it was happening."

One grieving widow I worked with told me the hardest days were after the condolence cards stopped coming. Others who have suffered the loss of a beloved find the hardest days are anniversaries when no one acknowledges that the date was once very special. Even recognizing of the anniversary of the day of death will be meaningful to the bereaved. Remember to be gentle and patient as your loved one finds his or her way in a new landscape.

Sky Blue Pink

Sometimes on your birthday, you spend the day thinking of "birth" days. You remember passionately the births of each of your children and how much in love you are with them. You know there is nothing that could ever separate you from the love you have for them and how blessed you are for their incredible gift of life. You think about your parents, and you wonder what it was like for them and your brothers the day you were born. A child's birth changes its mother's life in profound and everlasting ways that he or she will never fully understand. You must remember to tell your children their birth stories this year ...

Mostly you are grateful that you feel magically loved and cherished.

You weep a little thinking about last year's birthday. You reminded your mother to call all her children and grandchildren on their birthdays in her last year, but you were too humble to remind her of yours. You know it's not her fault she didn't remember. You should have told her ... Then you open the mail and you find a letter addressed to her. Coincidence? Perhaps. You decide that letter is her birthday greeting to you.

Later, you record "Happy Birthday" in the style of Mozart for your birthday buddies, (fitting since you were all *born on Mozart's birthday), then treat yourself to a dreamy massage. In the midst of post-massage bliss, you decide to make yourself an Angel food cake—the heavenly treat you always requested your mother make for you on your birthday. You liked how she would prop the pan upside down on a 7-Up bottle to cool it after she removed it from the oven. You use her angel food cake pan and flour sifter, and her "Fluffy Frosting" recipe, as dictated to you by her over the phone some years back.*

When he returns home from work, you head to your favorite Italian restaurant for dinner with your husband. On the way there you notice the color of the evening sky is vibrant pink and blue. You remember your colorblind father answering, "sky blue pink," when you would ask him what his favorite color was. You knew "sky blue pink" wasn't a real color. There was no crayon with that name in your box of sixty-four Crayola Crayons. But as you look in the sky today, you know that "sky blue pink" is indeed a real color.

Once at the restaurant, you order your meal and decide to have a glass of wine while you wait. You are not a regular wine drinker, and you realize after the first few sips that you forgot to eat lunch ... This wine is going to your head FAST! Dinner is particularly funny this evening as you giggle through your entree, giggle at yourself giggling, and giggle at your husband who is not giggling.

You return home and eat no less than one-fourth of your angel food cake, then begin to read the warm and fuzzy birthday greetings from your truly amazing family and friends. You are thankful for birthdays and "birth" days, birthday buddies and Mozart, Angel food cake and fluffy frosting, "sky blue pink" and wine, giggles and patient husbands, birthday calls from your children, and pages and pages of birthday greetings to enjoy. Mostly you are grateful that you feel magically loved and cherished, and you took the time to cherish yourself a little.

NOTES AND THOUGHTS

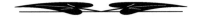

TIA AMDURER

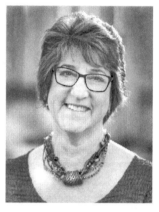

T ia Amdurer, LPC, enjoys sharing the art of storytelling whether it is through encouraging client narratives in her private therapy practice, writing newsletters, authoring articles, producing a documentary, or in her infamous annual holiday letter. Her first foray in publishing came in *Jack and Jill Magazine* in 1970 with an article titled "We Live in Kenya," detailing her childhood growing up in Africa with her family. After receiving her bachelor's degree in journalism and communications from the University of Delaware, she went on to a career in public relations in New York City. By 1990, she had moved with her husband and two children to Lakewood, Colorado, where she was a freelance writer and worked for several non-profits. In 2013 she produced an award-winning documentary film, *Heart and Sole: 20 years of Tap Extravaganza.*® Tia earned her MA in counseling from Regis University, worked in hospice for five years, and is grateful for the opportunity to provide therapy in grief and loss. Connect with Tia at:

TakeMyHandJourney@gmail.com

CHRIS RENAUD-COGSWELL

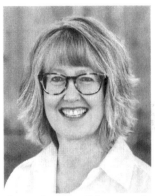

Chris Renaud-Cogswell is in high demand as an enthusiastic piano teacher for students with special needs. An advocate for accessibility, she guides her students in musical discovery and gives them the tools they need to succeed. A committed lifelong learner, she is currently pursuing continuing education at Metropolitan State University of Denver, exploring technology and designing teaching materials to engage all types of learners. Writing, both with words and with music, are the tools by which Chris processes the most painful and the most joyful events in her life. It is through her honest and creative voice that Chris enjoys sharing her eclectic observations on life. Chris is a native of Colorado where she enjoys more than anything, time spent with her brilliant, quirky children and beautiful grandchildren and searching for the perfect Mexican restaurant with Kevin, her devoted husband of 31 years. Connect with Chris at:

TakeMyHandJourney@gmail.com

REFERENCES

Abrahms, S. (2008). *Laughter yoga to improve health? It's no joke.* AARP.org. Retrieved from https://www.aarp.org/health/alternative-medicine/info-11-2008/laughter_yoga_to_improve.html.

Aging with Dignity. (2011). *Five wishes.* Tallahassee, FL: Aging with Dignity.

Dunn, H. (2009). *Hard choices for loving people: CPR, artificial feeding, comfort care, and the patient with a life-threatening illness.* Landsdowne, VA: A&A Publishers.

Ellers, K., Rikli, N., & Wright, H.N. (2006). *Grief following trauma.* Ellicott City, MD: International Critical Incident Stress Foundation, Inc.

Grassman, D. (Expert Panelist). (2017). *Soul injury: Liberating unmourned loss & unforgiven guilt.* Washington, DC: Hospice Foundation of America.

Karnes, B. (2014). *Gone from my sight.* Vancouver, WA: Barbara Karnes Books.

Mitchell, K. R. & Anderson, H. (1983). *All our losses, all our griefs.* Louisville, KY: Westminster John Knox Press.

Silk, S. & Goldman, B. (April 7, 2013). *How not to say the wrong thing. Los Angeles Times.* Retrieved from http://articles.latimes.com/2013/apr/07/opinion/la-oe-0407-silk-ring-theory-20130407

Wolfelt, A. (2015). *The paradoxes of mourning: Healing your grief with three forgotten truths.* Ft. Collins, CO: Companion Press.

RESOURCES

Preparation

AARP: www.aarp.org

Alzheimer's Association: www.alz.org

Michaels, L. and & Zilber, C. (2017). *Living in Limbo: Creating structure when someone you love is ill.* CreateSpace Independent Publishing Platform.

General Adult Grief

Attig, T. (2010). *How we grieve: Relearning the world.* Oxford, UK: Oxford University Press.

Coryell, D. M. (2007). *Good grief: Healing through the shadow of loss.* Rochester, VT: Healing Arts Press.

Deits, B. (2009). *Life after loss: A practical guide to renewing your life after experiencing major loss.* Cambridge, MA: Da Capo Lifelong Books.

Fumia, M. (2012). *Safe passage: Words to help the grieving.* Newberryport, MA: Conari Press.

James, J. W. & Cherry, F. (2009). *The grief recovery handbook.* New York, NY: Harper Perennial.

Kodanaz, R. B. (2013). *Living with loss, one day at a time.* Golden, CO: Fulcrum Publishing.

Komisky, P. (2007). *Getting back to life when grief won't heal.* New York, NY: McGraw-Hill.

Noel, B. & Blair, P. D. (2008). *I wasn't ready to say goodbye.* Naperville, IL: Sourcebooks.

Petrie, R. G. (2001). *Into the cave: When men grieve.* Oregon City, OR: One to another.

Rando, T. (1991). *How to go on living when someone you love dies.* London, UK: Bantam.

Smith, H. I. (2007). *ABC's of healthy grieving: A companion for everyday coping.* Notre Dame, IN: Ava Maria Press.

Tatelbaum, J. (2005). *You don't have to suffer.* Bloomington, IN: AuthorHouse.

Tatelbaum, J. (2008). *The courage to grieve: The classic guide to creative living, recovery and growth through grief.* New York, NY: William Morrow.

Wolfelt, A. (2001). *Healing your grieving heart.* Ft. Collins, CO: Companion Press.

Wolfelt, A. (2004). *Understanding your grief.* Ft. Collins, CO: Companion Press.

Death of a Spouse

Feinberg, L. (2013). *I'm grieving as fast as I can: How young widows and widowers can cope and heal.* Far Hills, NJ: New Horizon Press.

Heinlein, S. (1997). *When a life mate dies: Stories of love, loss and healing.* Minneapolis, MN: Fairview Press.

Schaefer, G. J. with Bekkers, T. (2011). *The widower's toolbox: Repairing your life after losing your spouse.* Far Hills, NJ: New Horizons Press.

Sharp , N. (2014). *Both sides now: A true story of love, loss and bold living.* Coral Gables, FL: Books & Books Press.

Staudacher, C. A. (1991). *Men and grief: A guide for men surviving the death of a loved one.* Oakland, CA: New Harbinger Publications, Inc.

Wolfelt, A. (2016). *When your soulmate dies*. Ft. Collins, CO: Companion Press.

Death of a Parent as an Adult Child

Brooks, J. (1999). *Midlife orphan: Facing life's changes now that your parents are gone*. New York, NY: Berkley Publishing Group.

Donnelly, K. F. (2015). *Recovering from the loss of a parent*. New York, NY: Open Road Distribution.

Levy , A. (2000). *The orphaned adult*. Cambridge, MA: Da Capo Press.

Marshall, F. (2009). *Losing a parent: A personal guide*. Cambridge, MA; Da Capo Press.

Meyers, D. (1997). *When parents die*. New York, NY: Penguin Books.

Wolfelt, A. (2002). *Healing the adult child's grieving heart: 100 practical ideas after your parent dies*. Ft. Collins, CO: Companion Press.

Religious-Themed/Contemplative

Brener, A. (2011). *Mourning & mitzvah*. Nashville, TN: Jewish Lights. (Jewish)

Dunn, B. & Leonard, K. (2004). *Through a season of grief.* New York, NY: Thomas Nelson. (Christian)

Levy, N. (2011). *To begin again*. New York, NY: Ballantine Books. (Jewish)

Lewis, C. S. (2009). *A grief observed*. New York, NY: HarperCollins. (Christian)

O'Donohue, J. (2008). *To bless the space between us: A book of blessings*. New York, NY: Harmony Books. (spiritual)

Rinpoche, S., Gafffney, P. & Harvey, A. (2009). *The Tibetan book of living and dying*. New York, NY: Harper Collins. (Buddhist)

Staudacher, C. A. (2011). *A time to grieve: Meditations for healing after the death of a loved one*. New York, NY: HarperOne.

Young Children

Brown, L.K. (1998). *When dinosaurs die*. New York, NY: Little, Brown.

Buscaglia, L. (1982). *The fall of Freddie the leaf*. Thorofare, NJ: Slack, Inc.

De Paola, T. (2000). *Nana upstairs and Nana downstairs*. New York, NY: GP Putnam & Sons.

Hanson, W. (2002). *The next place*. Golden Valley, MN: Waldman House Press, Inc.

Karst, P. (2000). *The invisible string*. Camarillo, CA: Devorss and Company.

Sabin, E. (2006). *The healing book: Facing the death and celebrating the life of someone you love*. China: Watering Can Press

Sharp, N. & Dodson, D. (2017). *Because the sky is everywhere*. Lithia Springs, GA: New Leaf Distributing Company.

Stenson, L., Stenson, A. & Friedersdorf, M. (2002). *Daddy, up and down: Sisters grieve the loss of their daddy*. Marceline, MO: Walsworth Publishing.

Thomas, P. (2001). *I miss you: A first look at death*. Hauppauge, NY: Barron's Educational Series.

Varley, S. (1992). *Badger's Parting Gifts*. New York, NY: HarperCollins.

Vigna, J. (1991). *Saying goodbye to daddy*. Morton Grove, IL: Albert Whitman & Co.

Welsh, P. (2005). *I wonder what you do on your first day in heaven*. Kirkwood, MO: Less is More Publishing.

CPSIA information can be obtained
at www.ICGtesting.com
Printed in the USA
FFOW03n1124050118
44367362-44070FF